D1562589

Pain and Suffering

Mission Statement of IASP Press

The International Association for the Study of Pain (IASP) is a non-profit, interdisciplinary organization devoted to understanding the mechanisms of pain and improving the care of patients with pain through research, education, and communication. The organization includes scientists and health care professionals dedicated to these goals. The IASP sponsors scientific meetings and publishes newsletters, technical bulletins, the journal *Pain,* and books.

The goal of IASP Press is to provide the IASP membership with timely, high-quality, low-cost publications relevant to the problem of pain. These publications are also intended to appeal to a wider audience of scientists and clinicians interested in the problem of pain.

Pain and Suffering

William K. Livingston, MD

Editor

Howard L. Fields, MD, PhD

Departments of Neurology and Physiology
University of California School of Medicine
San Francisco, California, USA

IASP PRESS • SEATTLE

Library of Congress Cataloging-in-Publication Data

Livingston, W. K. (William Kenneth), 1892–1966.
    Pain and Suffering / William K. Livingston ; editor, Howard L. Fields
      p. cm.
    Includes bibliographical references and index.
    ISBN 0-931092-24-8 (cloth)
    1. Livingston, W. K. (William Kenneth), 1892–1966. 2. Pain—Research—History.
I. Fields, Howard L. II. Title.
    [DNLM: 1. Livingston, W. K. (William Kenneth), 1892–1966.
2. Pain personal narratives. 3. Research personal narratives.   WL 704L787p 1998]
RB127.L48 1998
616' .047—dc21
[B]
DNLM/DLC
for Library of Congress   98-40341
                                                      CIP

Published by:

IASP Press
International Association for the Study of Pain
909 NE 43rd Street, Suite 306
Seattle, WA 98105-6020 USA
Fax: 206-547-1703

Printed in the United States of America

Contents

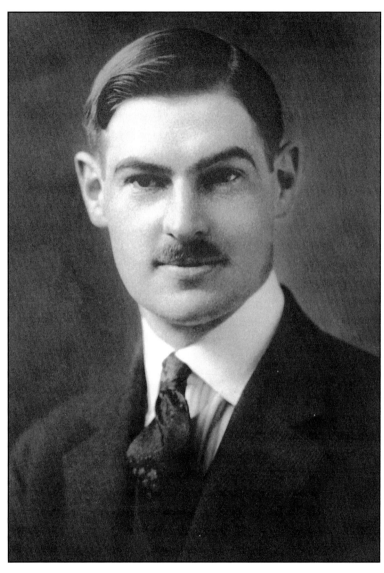

William K. Livingston
(1892–1966)

Foreword

This wonderful book is an adventure in ideas. The field of pain research and theory suddenly came alive in the second half of this century, full of new concepts and therapeutic approaches. Few persons contributed more to this breakthrough than William Kenneth Livingston. His earlier book, *Pain Mechanisms,* published in 1943, was the first major critique of the traditional specificity theory of pain. It marked the beginning of new ideas leading to the remarkable explosion of innovative research and new forms of treatment in recent decades. Livingston exposed the weaknesses of the traditional specificity theory with its concept of a straight-through transmission system and he began to explore new concepts: the temporal and spatial patterning of input, the importance of summation mechanisms, the dynamics of reverberatory circuits to account for persistent pathological pain states, the importance of the internuncial pools in the spinal cord in the gating of input, and the use of anesthetic blocks and stimulation techniques to modulate pain.

It was characteristic of Livingston to seek out every possible new approach to an understanding of pain. He invited promising young scientists to spend a year or two in his laboratory, with the idea that they should bring their skills to bear on the problem of pain and continue to work on it later in their careers. Happily, he accepted my request to spend a year with him. The year was extended to three years, and they were the most exciting of my career. It was my great privilege to work with Livingston as a postdoctoral fellow from 1954 to 1957.

Livingston chaired the Department of Surgery at the University of Oregon Medical School. He was convinced that every clinical department should have active research laboratories so that practicing physicians and research investigators could interact daily, exchange ideas, and stimulate new research and clinical approaches. Livingston's idea was particularly fruitful. He recognized that our knowledge of the pain signaling system was inadequate and he proposed stimulating the tooth pulp as a physiological source of pain signals throughout the brain. He believed that once the systems were known, their pharmacological, anatomical, and behavioral properties could be examined. As a result, a steady stream of papers on pain mechanisms appeared from the Department of Surgery.

In addition, Livingston organized weekly lunchtime pain seminars covering the full range of topics in biology and medicine. Their driving force was Livingston's capacity for enthusiasm and excitement. New ideas thrilled him the way new toys thrill small boys. His grin, his laugh, his enthusiasm were infectious. Discussion covered all the sensory modalities, the problem of memory in all its complexity, and clinical problems that provided valuable clues to the puzzle of pain. A small group, never more than fifteen persons, was invited to these seminars. They included selected staff from the clinical and basic departments of the medical school and physicians from "down the hill" (downtown Portland). These seminars were exciting, stimulating, and memorable.

Finally, Livingston established the Pain Clinic at the University Hospital, one of the first formal clinics to deal specifically with pain problems that could not be solved by other medical departments. Partway through my first year, Livingston invited me to attend the clinic. "It's time for scientists to get out of the laboratory and see what pain is really about," he told me. Held weekly, those clinic afternoons profoundly influenced my thinking about pain. I was exposed to the suffering caused by phantom-limb pain, heard despairing complaints of back pain and postherpetic neuralgia that failed to respond to surgery or drugs, saw patients weep because of the unremitting, burning pain of causalgia. Livingston treated those patients with a special compassion and kindness, and his brilliant questions (often asked for my benefit) revealed to me what he knew so well—that prolonged pain is debilitating, demoralizing, devastating. It grinds people down and makes life a burden. Patients doubt themselves and think they must be crazy if so many operations and treatments do not take their pain away. And, Livingston pointed out to me, in their frustration over their inability to help the patient, physicians sometimes reinforced that view with great psychological harm to the patient.

Bill Livingston was a big, open, warm, wonderful person. Born in Wisconsin in 1892 and raised in Wisconsin and Oregon, he received his medical training at Harvard Medical School and did a residency in surgery at the Massachusetts General Hospital. In 1922 he returned to the West Coast to set up a private practice. To get his practice under way, he served as a state medical officer on worker's compensation cases. Here he encountered cases of causalgia, whiplash injury, phantom-limb pain, and myriad baffling pain cases that simply could not be understood in terms of the traditional textbook story of pain mechanisms. He discovered the work of Weir Mitchell, who became his model of a great physician, and he knew all of Mitchell's published work almost from memory. When World War II broke out, Livingston joined the navy and soon reached the rank of commander. He requested work on peripheral nerve injury and soon became head of the Oakland Naval Hospital's division on peripheral nerve injuries. After publication of his book, *The Clinical Aspects of Visceral Neurology,* in 1935, he steadily contributed to the literature on pain. All his wisdom, experience, and compassionate fascination with pain were integrated into *Pain Mechanisms,* published in 1943.

Pain Mechanisms received good reviews but little real recognition beyond lip service. It simply wasn't understood. The 1940s and 1950s were the heyday of specificity, when textbooks and research entrenched the concept that the degree of pain experience is proportional to the extent of injury and that the way to block pain is to cut pain nerves and pathways. Despite lack of recognition, Livingston persisted in his teaching, research, and writing. He knew he was on the right track and he kept his eye solidly on what he believed was true: pain is complex; it is determined by interactions of inputs at all levels of the central nervous system; and it should be treated by modulating the input rather than cutting nerves.

Because they were so far ahead of his time, Bill Livingston's ideas tended to isolate him. But his devoted clinical colleagues and the postdoctoral fellows who worked with him helped him through times of doubt and occasional despair. His greatest source of joy and support was his family. His charming and delightful wife Ruth gave him love and a peaceful home life. In addition to his work, he excelled in everything he undertook: archery, horsemanship, fishing, wrestling (in his youth), and gardening. He played the clarinet well and often invited friends to his home to play chamber music. His two sons, Kenneth and Robert, were special sources of pride. He took enormous pleasure in Ken's capacity to combine clinical medicine and research and in Bob's work on the functions of the brainstem reticular formation.

Livingston began writing *Pain and Suffering* in 1956. After his retirement in 1958, he and Ruth moved to the glorious Metolius country in eastern Oregon, where he raised plants and became an expert potter, making his own glazes out of local stones. He also worked hard on this new book on pain, which he had planned and organized for years. Pain, he argues in this book, is a transactional process involving continuing interactions and feedback loops among all parts of the nervous system.

On March 21, 1966, Bill Livingston died peacefully in his sleep. Along with his other papers, the book manuscript was held in safe-keeping by his son Bob and later by the Oregon Health Sciences University Library. Happily, John Liebeskind acquired the manuscript for the History of Pain Collection that he and medical historian Marcia Meldrum were developing for the Louise M. Darling Biomedical Library at UCLA. Now we are enriched through its publication by IASP Press. Livingston's book is as exciting and inspiring now as it was when he wrote it.

Pain and Suffering is a monument to a great scientist and human being. I recall when he sat in my office one Friday afternoon, about to leave for the weekend. He had been writing since 5 A.M. that day—his usual routine—but had decided the material was bad and had torn it all up. He was wistful and a little depressed. He asked how my research was coming along. Happily, it had been a good week, and Bill beamed to hear about our new evidence for a brainstem system that exerts continuous descending inhibitory control over pain-signaling input. He cheered up considerably. "You know, Ron," he said, "science is like a community hat into which each person contributes a little bit. Some people's work is like adding a few pennies; other people contribute nickels and dimes. Some hotshot may throw in the occasional quarter." He laughed and his eyes twinkled. "We never really know how much we contribute," he continued. "History will tell that."

History already shows how great indeed was Bill Livingston's contribution to the field of pain, to the alleviation of human suffering—more than he ever dreamed.

RONALD MELZACK, PHD
McGill University
Montreal, Quebec, Canada

Historical Note

The original manuscript of *Pain and Suffering* is in the John C. Liebeskind History of Pain Collection at the Louise M. Darling Biomedical Library at UCLA. How the book came to UCLA and how it was almost lost and then was rediscovered by John Liebeskind is a story in itself.

William K. Livingston worked on *Pain and Suffering* for nearly twenty years; he had just completed what he thought would be a final draft when he died in 1966. He had been pleased with the manuscript and had begun to talk about publishers. His sons, Robert and Kenneth, kept the final draft with his other papers. Robert compiled an index of the papers, but he and Kenneth were busy with their own careers and did not have the time to edit the manuscript for publication. After Kenneth's death his widow, Katherine, found the papers in the family home at Camp Sherman, Oregon, and donated them to the Oregon Health Sciences University (OHSU) Library. The library lacked sufficient funds to process the papers, so the manuscript remained filed away and almost forgotten.

In 1992 John C. Liebeskind, professor of psychology at UCLA, began the History of Pain Project, a major effort to document the history of the pain field in the twentieth century. He conducted oral history interviews and located and preserved the written records of the most influential investigators and clinicians. When he interviewed Ronald Melzack in 1993, Melzack spoke warmly of his mentor, Livingston, and suggested to Liebeskind that his papers, including an unpublished manuscript, might have been preserved. Following this lead, Liebeskind began to search for members of the Livingston family. In 1995 he made contact with Robert Livingston, who explained that the papers had been donated to OHSU. Robert gave Liebeskind a copy of his index, several photographs, and a bust of Livingston, which is now on display in the biomedical library at UCLA.

Liebeskind contacted Katherine Livingston and Heather Rosenwinkel, the history of medicine librarian at OHSU, and arranged a loan of the Livingston papers to UCLA. We were fascinated by these papers, which included interesting correspondence on the subject of pain, case histories of nerve injuries from World War II, the notes of

Livingston's visits to pain laboratories around the country, and the manuscript of *Pain and Suffering*. We immediately recognized the importance of this book.

Liebeskind's enthusiasm for the Livingston materials convinced the family and Rosenwinkel that UCLA would be an appropriate home for them as an integral part of the History of Pain Collection. This unique collection would include the papers of John Bonica, founder of the International for the Study of Pain, Dutch surgeon and pain theorist Willem Noordenbos, and John Liebeskind himself, as well as forty of Liebeskind's oral history interviews with pain scientists and clinicians. The official transfer occurred in spring 1997. Shortly afterward, Liebeskind learned that he had terminal throat cancer. He devoted his last months to working with me to ensure the continuation and growth of the History of Pain Collection.

Among the projects we discussed was the publication of *Pain and Suffering*. John Loeser, chair of the American Pain Society's 20th Anniversary Task Force, had asked for suggestions for the commemorative celebration—perhaps a book of important papers on pain? Liebeskind saw the opportunity; he and I agreed to propose publication of the Livingston manuscript to the task force. The APS and IASP Press also recognized the quality and importance of *Pain and Suffering*, which is in a sense the legacy of two men who greatly influenced the field of pain research and treatment.

MARCIA MELDRUM, PhD
Department of History
University of California at Los Angeles

Preface

On behalf of the American Pain Society, I am pleased and privileged to present this previously unpublished manuscript by William K. Livingston. Publication of this insightful and inspiring book resulted from the dedicated efforts of many persons, principal among them the late John Liebeskind, APS Historian Marcia Meldrum, Editor Howard Fields, and John Loeser, chairman of the APS Twentieth Anniversary Task Force. The generous support of APS corporate sponsors helped fund publication of *Pain and Suffering*.

William Livingston was a forward-thinking, caring clinician and scientist whose contributions to our understanding of pain and suffering have been grossly underappreciated. As Ronald Melzack indicates in his Foreword, Livingston's ideas and concepts about pain mechanisms and modulation were well ahead of their time and simply not always understood or appreciated. I hope that publication of his manuscript, for which APS is indebted to the Livingston family, finally assigns to Livingston the recognition he richly deserves.

The interesting story of how Livingston's manuscript became the book you now hold is summarized in the Historical Note by Marcia Meldrum. The APS is grateful to John Liebeskind and Marcia Meldrum for advancing this historically and intellectually valuable manuscript as appropriate to the celebration of the twentieth anniversary of the APS. Livingston's "final draft" was far from being ready for publication when it was discovered. This book would not have reached print without the invaluable editorial contributions of Howard Fields. All who read and enjoy this exceptional book are indebted to Dr. Fields for his editorial skill, industry, and enthusiasm for this project. The APS also extends a special thank you to the IASP Press for its invaluable assistance and dedication in bringing this project to completion. Listed on the following page are the corporations whose financial support enabled the American Pain Society to provide complimentary copies of this outstanding book to all APS members attending the twentieth-anniversary meeting.

G.F. GEBHART, PhD
President, American Pain Society, 1997–98

For their support for the publication of *Pain and Suffering*,
the American Pain Society thanks:

Abbott Laboratories
Algos Pharmaceutical Corporation
Endo Pharmaceuticals Inc.
Faulding Laboratories
Janssen Pharmaceutica
Knoll Pharmaceutical Company
Ortho-McNeil Pharmaceutical
The Purdue Frederick Company
Roxane Laboratories
Searle

Introductory Note

Receiving this manuscript by William K. Livingston more than thirty years after his death was a deeply moving experience for me. Delving into it immediately brought to mind the image of uncovering sunken treasure. I would like to thank the Livingston family for sharing this treasure with us. As discussed in the historical note, John Liebeskind and Marcia Meldrum of UCLA were instrumental in bringing this manuscript to the attention of the American Pain Society and IASP Press. Because this book is an important historical document, it is fitting that it is being published on the twentieth anniversary of the APS.

In this semiautobiographical work Livingston reveals to us a unique perspective that speaks across time. He becomes our guide and colleague, a person whose experience with pain patients rivals that of the historical giants in the field: S. Weir Mitchell, René Leriche, and Sir Thomas Lewis. This is a colleague whose infectious enthusiasm, inquisitive mind, and total dedication to understanding pain draws us to him and to his brilliantly described patients. One can only imagine the delight of discussing a puzzling case with him.

Two key events in 1965 spurred the study of pain as an independent medical and scientific field: the establishment of the multidisciplinary pain clinic at the University of Washington by John J. Bonica and the publication of Melzack and Wall's gate-control hypothesis. Livingston's manuscript, completed the same year, documents that he, too, was at the forefront in the development of the field. We learn that his interest was piqued by clinical experiences as a surgical resident at Harvard and during World War II as a surgeon at Oak Knoll Naval Hospital in Oakland, California. During his tenure as chair of surgery at the University of Oregon Medical School he not only led one of the first multidisciplinary pain clinics, he gathered a team of basic scientists to study the neurobiology of pain. He also traveled to the laboratories and clinical offices of leading scientists and physicians around the world to observe and discuss their work. It is difficult to imagine a more effective and dedicated leader for the field of pain research and treatment.

Although our understanding of the neurobiology of pain has far surpassed that of Livingston's era, his clinical and animal observations anticipated many trends in current pain research. These include the role of multiple ascending pathways in pain perception, the powerful influence of descending pain-modulating pathways, the importance of central sensitization, the role of inflammation in activating visceral nociceptors, and the importance of learning, attention, and expectation on perceived pain intensity.

A recurring theme in this book—and I suspect a factor that prompted Livingston to write it—is his struggle to apply his unique clinical and scientific knowledge to uncovering the fundamental nature of pain. In the final chapter we get a glimpse of the direction he was headed through the device of his fanciful "mind-body" debate between philosopher and physiologist. To Livingston, pain is apparently best thought of as the subjective perception that accompanies an appetitive state. This state arises from neuronal activity in aversive circuits of the brain, including those discovered by Olds and his colleagues in the mid-fifties. These circuits are integrative systems that have evolved to enhance the survival of the species. Livingston's final point seems to be that the specificity of the pain sensory system lies not in nociceptive primary afferents nor in the pain and temperature pathways projecting to somatosensory cortex, but in the aversive systems of the "transactional core." This concept presaged the "affective motivational" system described by Melzack and Casey in a paper published only two years after Livingston died.[1]

Although this book is historically significant, it offers much more than a glimpse of the past. It is a guide for those of us who constantly strive to improve our clinical skills. Livingston was an astute clinical observer who endeavored to improve the treatment of his patients through deeper understanding of the neural mechanisms of pain. Curiosity coupled with compassion and concern guided his patient descriptions. If something about a patient didn't fit with his mechanistic understanding, he would seek a better explanation by using animal models to explore the question. In the final analysis, however, everything revolved around the patient's reported experience. Consequently, the clinical material in this book is uniquely valuable. Livingston's observations were tempered by both vast clinical experience and insa-

---

[1]Melzack R, Casey KL. Sensory, motivational, and central control determinants of pain: a new conceptual model. In D Kenshalo (Ed): *The Skin Senses*. Springfield, IL: Charles Thomas, 1968, pp 423–439.

tiable curiosity about underlying neural mechanisms. This approac
at once informative and inspirational. It views the ideal practice o
medicine as just that—a practice, a life-long exercise in self-education.
This book can serve that end for all of us.

HOWARD L. FIELDS, PHD
University of California
at San Francisco

from experiments performed on animals. But there are limits to the extent we can rely upon such inferences. It seems reasonable to assume that experimentally induced pains experienced by animals may be similar to those of humans because the higher animals respond reflexively and behaviorally much as humans do to the noxious stimuli customarily employed in the research laboratory. But there are good reasons to doubt that an animal's pain is subject to exactly the same psychological influences that affect a human, and I have been able to find no evidence that an animal ever suffers from major causalgia or any of the other "pathological" pain states that cause humans the most terrible forms of pain. Furthermore, we already know that inferences drawn from experimental studies conducted on animals deeply asleep under a general anesthetic drug may have nothing to do with pain as human patients know it.

Perhaps the most serious obstacle to any study of pain in the research laboratory is that a pain represents a dynamic transaction occurring in that mysterious embodiment of brain activity that is called the "mind." To the extent possible, scientists usually avoid using the word "mind" because, until they know more about how a brain can function as a mind, the word will continue to suggest that old bugaboo of a mind-body dichotomy. But whether investigators elect to deal with pain as a sensation, a perception, or a symptom, they cannot avoid the fact that no human being uses the word "pain" to designate a subjective experience unless its obnoxious qualities are consciously perceived and recognized as such. (Bluntly stated, the task of the laboratory worker is to identify all the factors contributing to an intangible transaction occurring within an equally intangible mind.) It is no wonder then that each individual investigator tends to focus on the aspect of pain that is most apparent from the unique point of view predetermined by the investigator's special training and professional interests. He may be aware of other aspects of pain but usually ignores them, either because he lacks the tools and techniques with which to analyze them or he considers it hopeless to try to investigate all of them simultaneously. Thus, the study of pain has progressed by a process of "dissection" with the resulting accumulation of a vast literature relating to the biological, sociological, philosophical, physiological, psychological, and clinical aspects of pain along with discrepant definitions for the word that reveal the biases of their originators.

I know of no better way to appreciate the confused state of our present knowledge about this general subject than to collect all the available definitions of "pain" found in dictionaries and textbooks in the various fields of science and philosophy. A critical examination of such a collection might bring to mind the old tale of the three blind men, each of whom attempted to describe an elephant in terms of the one part of the animal's body he had touched. The critic might then come to feel, as I do, that each definition, like each of the three descriptions of the elephant, may be true enough as far as it goes and yet may fall far short of defining a dynamic whole.

This introduction is not the place to list numerous definitions, but perhaps I can indicate the divergence of opinion by giving a brief sketch of two opposing interpretations of pain. According to the definitions listed in *Webster's International Dictionary*, it should be permissible to use this word to designate any kind of unpleasant subjective experience whether it originates in the body or in the mind and whether it is mild discomfort or extreme torture. This broad definition, which makes pain the antithesis of pleasure and which does not distinguish between physical pain and such emotions as grief and anxiety, is based on the teachings of all the great philosophers and has become commonplace in our literature and daily language. Many people reject this interpretation and would be inclined to say that what the dictionary is defining is not pain but some affective state of the mind such as "suffering" or "unpleasantness."

Here is an alternative interpretation that has received considerable support in the past: pain is a "primary sensory modality." It is one of the special body senses, like sight or hearing. Pain has its own specifically adapted peripheral receptor, its own conduction pathway in the spinal cord, and its own perceptual center in the sensory area of the cerebral cortex of the brain. The point-to-point connection between the site of noxious stimulation and the appropriate part of the sensory cortex ensures that the "sensation" of pain will be an exact replica of the external stimulus configuration. Thus, the severity of the pain is always directly proportional to stimulus intensity and any apparent deviation from the constancy of this relationship must be attributed to the person's psychological reaction to the pain.

I am not attributing this latter interpretation to any particular source but I think it summarizes most of the teachings on which I based my original concept of pain as it was formulated a half-century ago. At the time I could see more clearly than now how silly it was of the philosophers to confuse pain with suffering. I could understand how important it was for a physician to be able to distinguish between a patient's pain and his psychological reaction to it because these two components of suffering required different modes of treatment. I knew that patients sometimes exaggerated their complaints of pain but I assumed that when I had identified the cause of their pain I could tell from the nature of the organic lesion whether their pain complaints were real or due to psychological factors.

When I began to practice as a surgeon these assumptions seemed to hold true for the ordinary run of contusions, lacerations, and fractures that I treated. But every once in a while I would be baffled by my inability to detect any organic lesion to account for a patient's complaints of disabling pain. The case might be one of posttraumatic headache, a back strain, or the so-called "whiplash" injury to the neck. In the absence of any demonstrable source for the pain it was easy to assume that these patients must be neurasthenic, hysterical, or malingering, particularly in cases that involved the question of monetary compensation. I regret to say that in the early years of practice I probably made such diagnoses too readily and talked too glibly of such things as "psychogenic pain" and "psychic overlay." But then it happened that for some eight years I served part-time as a medical examiner for the Oregon State Industrial Accident Commission. In this assignment I encountered dozens of similar cases. I was impressed by the similarity of the complaints in each type of injury and by their numbers. There were also many cases of both major and minor causalgia and of phantom limb pain. I found that my co-examiners accepted such pain complaints as real and disabling, although they were rather vaguely ascribed to "nerve irritation." But in the medical reports of these state cases, written by the patients' attending physicians, I found repeated denials of the reality of the patients' pains and recurring diagnoses of hysteria and malingering in cases in which I felt sure such diagnoses were not justifiable. And I finally decided that there must be something wrong with the concept of pain we doctors acquire in medical school and that *any* mechanistic concept of pain might handicap a physician's efforts to understand what might be called "pathological" types of pain or the most serious human pain problems.

It was to suggest a more dynamic concept of pain that I wrote the little book entitled *Pain Mechanisms* that the Macmillan Company published in 1943. But even as that book was being written, I was aware of the need for more experimental evidence to support my speculative and unorthodox interpretations. In the hope of securing such evidence I joined, in 1947, with a group of faculty members of the University of Oregon Medical School to conduct a team investigation of human pain problems in our clinics and research laboratories. In the eleven years we worked together, members of the team published many individual pieces of research in various professional journals. But no one has yet volunteered to report our seminar discussions and the impressions of the team as a whole. My colleagues have urged me to undertake this assignment. I have begged off because I felt that to do justice to the task I would have to write a type of "review" that would be expected to cite chapter, verse, and line for each reference and to use a scientific terminology that might render what I wanted to say inaccessible to all but an esoteric group of experts. I wanted to deal with pain not as a scientifically established entity but as an "evolving idea" that could be expected to evolve still further as we learned more about how a brain can function as a mind. In writing about it I wished to avoid any pose of authority or any involvement in arguments with friends who might not agree with my interpretations.

Several years ago, Alan Gregg, a friend, suggested that I might best accomplish these purposes by writing a simple story of my own efforts to formulate a concept of pain, a story that might be flexible enough to apply to both pathological pain and experimentally induced types of pain. This suggestion appealed to me. I thought it might be rather fun and relatively easy to identify the successive changes in my concept of pain that evolved from my clinical experience and exposure to conflicting opinion. But all the fun went out of the task long ago and now, years and barrels of discarded manuscript later, I am not pleased with what I have written. As I reread parts of the story it seems to me that I alternate between sounding hopelessly naive and sounding like a stuffed shirt, and I seem to be unable to modify either impression.

The first chapter sketches in the background for the formulation of my original "push-button" concept of pain; then, with all its faults and for whatever it may be worth, the story of the evolving idea follows.

1

The Interpretive Background
For a Concept of Pain

This is to be a story about an "evolving idea," a concept of pain that was first formulated fifty years ago when I was a medical student. To understand its original assumptions one ought to know something about the interpretive climate that existed in the early years of the twentieth century. The nineteenth century had witnessed a tremendous advance in all branches of science and I doubt that there has ever been a time, before or since, when scientists felt more confident that they were on the right track in their efforts to account for natural phenomena. All nature was supposed to conform to the Newtonian laws of physics and the atom was held to be the ultimate manifestation of matter. Some ninety elements had been identified and arranged in the orderly sequence of an atomic table. In the physics laboratory, these elements could be pushed about by various forms of energy and in the chemistry laboratory they could be united in various combinations that might alter their outward appearance, but nothing could ever alter their elemental nature. It is true that a few men, possessed with unusual insight, had begun to question these basic assumptions, but the "revolution" in interpretive thought which their investigations were to initiate had not yet started. I know that this was so because for two years before I entered medical school, I taught courses in physics and chemistry to high school students and was supremely confident that the "facts" I was helping them learn were well-established "truths" rather than assumptions. I can remember telling my students that the greatest joke in the history of science was the foolish dream of the alchemists that means might be found for transmuting base metals into gold.

In this same period medical practice was in the final phase of its "horse-and-buggy" stage as an "art" and beginning to lay claims of being a "science." The monumental contributions of such men as Virchow, Pasteur, Koch, and Ehrlich were stimulating intensive effort by scientists to identify the cellular changes characteristic of each disease, to discover the specific microbe causing each one, and to find the specific drug that would destroy the microorganism without doing too much harm to its host. Indeed, the early years of the twentieth century might be called the "era of specificity" because of the emphasis on the effort to establish a direct connection between the single cause and its effect.

It was in this era that I began my four years of medical school training. It was probably fortunate that I began then because medical faculties were much less fussy about admissions and there was so much less for the student to learn than there is now. Nor was there any reason for the student to doubt that the facts he was learning were well-established truths. I remember that we students were often reminded to "stick to the facts," "keep your feet on the ground," and "avoid arm-chair philosophizing." In the laboratories we spent much time over our microscopes examining normal tissue sections and all kinds of pathological specimens. In the clinic we were discouraged from making more than one diagnosis for a single case, and in the autopsy room we were urged to find the single cause of death. One might almost have reduced our teachings to a formula: "One patient = one diagnosis; one microbe = one disease; one drug = one therapeutic effect; and one death = one cause." Of course I am exaggerating, for we had many wise men among our teachers, but the general emphasis on specificity was surely there.

Much the same was true for the teachings we received about the anatomy and physiology of the central nervous system. The model for this system was a telephone exchange that automatically transmitted intact messages from one station to another over the long fiber tracts. Each function of the body was assumed to be under the control of one or more special "centers" within the great masses of gray matter, and the motor output was depicted as descending from cortical levels through a hierarchy of functional levels to reach the muscles and glands of the body. In much the same fashion the sensory input from the body was supposed to be carried by the long fiber tracts directly to the appropriate receiving centers in the sensory areas of the cerebral cortex. The

*. . . it should not be surprising that
my original concept of pain was
mechanistic and rigid. I learned to draw a
diagram of this "three-neuron pain-pathway"
and I believed that I understood how it
functioned as well as I understood the
operation of the simple electrical circuit
that rang my front doorbell.*

functional unit of the nervous system was the single neuron, which fired or failed to fire in an "all-or-none" fashion, so that a sensory message coming in from the periphery passed directly from one neuron on to the next to reach a perceptual level, thus ensuring that the "sensation" would represent an exact replica of the external stimulus configuration. The building block from which the entire nervous system was thought to have evolved was the simple reflex for which the relationship between a stimulus and its response was almost as direct and immediate as a knee jerk, and voluntary movement could be referred to as merely a glorified reflex.

In this interpretive climate it should not be surprising that my original concept of pain was mechanistic and rigid. According to the assumptions of the "punctate theory" I learned that there were only "four modalities of cutaneous sensibility"—touch, pain, heat, and cold. I remember that in the physiology laboratory I mapped out a mosaic of the four kinds of "skin spot," each of which produced one of these sensations following the application of mechanical pressure. I assumed that beneath each pain spot must be located a specifically adapted "pain fiber." This fiber was said to be nonmyelinated and to have naked terminals, a type of fiber now classified as a "C fiber." I learned to identify these pain fibers under a microscope and found them in tissue sections taken from all parts of the human body. I understood that a pain fiber could be activated by any kind of a stimulus—mechanical, electrical, thermal, or chemical—but only when such a stimulus reached an intensity that began to damage the tissue cells. The impulses thus set up in the pain fiber were carried into the spinal cord, where they first served to initiate a train of protective reflexes, and then ascended in the specialized "pain and temperature" tract to the thalamus and from there were carried to the somatic sensory area of the cerebral cortex where they gave rise to the sensation of pain. I learned to draw a diagram of this "three-neuron pain-pathway" and I believed that I understood how it functioned as well as I understood the operation of the simple electrical circuit that rang my front doorbell. All one had to do to elicit pain was to press the right button at the periphery and the pain bell would inevitably ring in consciousness. The harder the button was pressed, the louder the bell would ring.

In this book I shall hereafter refer to that original formulation as my "push-button" concept of pain because of its mechanistic features. I am not using that designation in a derogatory sense, because there is much truth in its assumptions; but as the following story is intended to show, it had certain shortcomings.

2

Opening a Colostomy

In June 1920, I graduated from Harvard Medical School and immediately began a two-year surgical internship in the Massachusetts General Hospital. The surgical service on which I was enrolled as a "house pupil" was organized in a ladder-like series of progressions up which an intern moved at three-month intervals. At each step up, the intern took on assignments involving greater responsibility. On the top rung of this ladder was the "Senior" in his final three months of training, who was held responsible by the Resident Surgeon and the Visiting Staff for the performances of all the other interns on the service, much as the captain of a naval vessel is held responsible for the behavior of his crew. Next in line of command was the "Junior," whose functions corresponded to those of an executive officer. At the bottom of the ladder was the newly arrived intern. He was called the "Pup" and, as the name implies, he was at the beck and call of all the other interns on the service. Each morning the Pup reported to the Junior and was given a list of his duties for that day. The list was usually long and included such menial tasks as cutting plaster casts, administering subpectoral infusions of salt solution to ill patients, passing catheters, and performing routine laboratory tests. The Pup rarely managed to complete his list of duties for the day. When he did manage to get them all done before midnight, he could be sure that more tasks would be wished off on him by other interns.

The event I wish to describe took place during my third week of service as Pup, when I was just beginning to get over my feeling of awe in the new environment. It started when the Junior handed me my list of assignments for that day. As I glanced over it, an unfamiliar item caught my eye. It recorded a patient's name and room number, after which appeared the cryptic notation, "open colostomy." I knew quite a bit about this particular patient because I had recorded his history and physical findings a few days previously when he had been admitted to the hospital complaining of severe cramping pains in his lower abdomen. Subsequently, a staff surgeon had explored this man's belly and had found the cause of his trouble to be a large growth involving the terminal portion of his large intestine. During this operation I had been privileged to hold a retractor so that I was able to see the mass, which the surgeon believed was cancerous. I had assumed that this mass had blocked the fecal stream and that the efforts of the colon to force its contents past this obstruction had caused the patient's cramping pains. At this operation the surgeon had not attempted to remove the cancerous mass but had set the stage for its subsequent excision by bringing up a loop of transverse colon and anchoring it in the belly wall so that a portion of the loop protruded externally. It was my understanding that as soon as the wound had sealed off around the exposed loop, an opening could be made into the loop that would permit the bowel content to escape through it. This vent would not only be expected to relieve the man of his cramping pains but would also permit a cleansing of the interior of the colon so as to reduce the chances of secondary infection of the wound after the second operation for removal of the cancerous mass.

Based on this understanding of the case, I had some notion of what the instruction "open colostomy" must mean. My difficulty was that I had never seen a colostomy opened and I had no notion of how to go about it. I ventured to say this to the Junior and to ask for specific instructions. "There is nothing to it!" he told me, "All you have to do is to burn a good hole in the loop—not a 'medical' hole but a good, big 'surgical' hole." I asked him what I should use to do the burning. He directed me to a certain closet near the surgeries where I would find a plumber's blowtorch. He went on, "If you haven't brains enough to light the thing, get someone to light it for you. Heat the soldering iron until it turns cherry-red in color, not white-hot, just a bright red, and then use the iron to burn an ample hole in the colon." I asked him which operating room I should use in carrying out the burning procedure. He fairly barked at me, "Don't take that patient anywhere. Take

. . . the Junior went with me to the closet to get the blowtorch. He lit it and started the soldering iron heating. It was beginning to glow a dull red when we walked into the patient's room carrying the blowtorch, roaring full blast, between us.

the blowtorch to his room and do the burning right there in his bed." I ventured to ask one more question: "What anesthetic should I give him before I burn him?" This time, his patience exhausted, the Junior almost exploded, "Hell, Bill, he won't need any anesthetic. He won't feel a damned thing!"

During this exchange my enthusiasm for opening a colostomy had steadily fallen and this last comment finished off the last of it. I was almost abject in pleading, "If you would just show me how the thing is done this one time, I will gladly open the next hundred colostomies for you." By now, thoroughly exasperated and grumbling about my "lack of guts" and how busy he was, the Junior went with me to the closet to get the blowtorch. He lit it and started the soldering iron heating. It was beginning to glow a dull red when we walked into the patient's room carrying the blowtorch, roaring full blast, between us. The patient reared up from his pillow and demanded to know what we were going to do with "that thing." My companion calmly told him to lie down; that we would use it to burn open his colostomy but he would feel nothing of the burning process. The patient did not reply, just lay staring at the blowtorch. I could see that he had no more confidence in the Junior's assurances than I had. While I removed the surgical dressings to expose the colon loop, the Junior moistened a large towel with water and draped it over the man's belly wall so that only the loop of gut was exposed like a red rosette within its folds. By this time the soldering iron was beginning to glow with a nice cherry-red color. As the Junior brought the glowing iron toward him, the patient again reared up from his pillow, his eyes staring and his fists tightly clenched at his sides, as if he was trying to steel himself to endure some agonizing torture.

The contact of the hot iron with the moist flesh gave rise to a sizzling sound. A thin wisp of smoke rose from the iron and the room began to fill with the stench of burning flesh. A hole appeared in the center of the loop and some fluid, mixed with gas, burbled out. The hole rapidly enlarged as the burning progressed, until it was about an inch in diameter. There was very little oozing of blood from its charred margins when the burning had been completed, and the surgical dressings were reapplied.

Every detail of this scene is vivid in my memory. I can almost imagine I can hear the sizzle, see the smoke, and smell the acrid odor. Most clearly of all I remember the look of fear and revulsion on the patient's face as he watched the red-hot iron coming toward him and then the astonishing change in his expression as the burning began. Then he smiled, relaxed, and lay back on his pillow, having felt nothing whatever of the burning process. I think that I was as surprised as he that he felt no pain, and I am sure it took me longer to relax my sweaty fists. I had done my best to appear nonchalant during the whole procedure as if it were a commonplace event, as indeed it was for anyone but a greenhorn like me.

First experiences always make a deep impression. Every physician remembers his first day in the anatomy dissecting room, the first autopsy he saw being done, and the first cesarean section he watched a surgeon perform. I can recall many details of each of these firsts in my training period but none of them made the impression on me that this opening a colostomy did. Perhaps I was better prepared for the other firsts in that what I saw corresponded more closely to what I had expected to see.

These other invasions of the human body, gruesome though they might appear to the uninitiated, carried with them no implication of suffering. The dead can feel no pain, and the woman I had seen undergoing the cesarean section had been deeply asleep under a general anesthetic. In contrast, the colostomy patient was fully awake and in full possession of his senses. He had obviously expected to be subjected to the torture of a burning, yet the burning had elicited no withdrawal reflexes and the patient had smiled while the wall of his colon was being destroyed by a red-hot iron.

Of course, I should have known that this patient would feel no pain because it was a fact long known to medical science that the internal organs can be cut, crushed, or burned without causing a fully conscious person any pain. I must have heard this fact stated by one or more of my instructors during the four years spent in medical school. But if so, the telling of it had made little impression on me until its truth had been demonstrated in this dramatic fashion. I could think of little else for days afterward, but it was neither the drama of the event nor the fact itself that was so disturbing to me. I could have accepted the fact in the same uncritical attitude I had displayed toward most of my medical instruction if only I could have fitted it into my push-button concept of pain.

After the lapse of more than forty-five years it would be foolish to pretend that I can now reconstruct exactly what went on in my mind at the time. But I do know that it was a period of real mental distress and I can guess at a few of the questions that were causing it. This patient had entered the hospital seeking relief from cramping pains in his abdomen. I had assumed that these pains originated in his intestine. I was sure that I had seen typical "pain fibers" under my microscope when examining stained sections of human intestine. The presumptive evidence was that the patient's colon *did* contain pain fibers that had already demonstrated their ability to ring the pain bell to warn him that something was seriously wrong inside his belly. But if so, why had the bell failed to ring while the colon was being burned with a red-hot iron?

Perhaps I had been wrong in thinking that the internal organs were supplied with pain fibers but if so, how could his cramping pains be accounted for? Perhaps there was more than one kind of pain fiber with different physiological properties. Maybe the kind supplied to the internal organs had a different threshold for activation than the kind supplied to skin or possibly was uniquely adapted to respond to only one kind of stimulation. The only kind of pain fiber my instructors had told me about was the one activated by any stimulus of sufficient intensity to threaten damage to tissue cells and which gave rise to pain sensation that was directly proportional to stimulus intensity. If there were other kinds I would have to reorganize my push-button concept and give up my notion of a "specific" pain fiber.

There was at least one other possible solution to my problem that may not have occurred to me at the time but that I considered later. Perhaps I had been wrong in thinking of pain in terms of my diagram of a three-neuron pain pathway in which the ringing of the pain bell could be achieved by activating a single pain fiber at the periphery. Maybe the pain bell would ring only when many pain fibers had been simultaneously activated. I knew that the population of pain fibers was much more dense in skin than in intestine, and this might mean that any noxious stimulus applied to skin would activate many pain fibers simultaneously while the same internal organ would activate too few to give rise to pain sensation. Perhaps violent peristaltic contractions of the gut served to activate the proper number of pain fibers while burning with a hot iron failed to do so.

Whatever my thought processes at the time, I remember that I soon stopped talking about the problem with the other interns because neither they nor I could understand why I allowed myself to become so steamed up about it. I wanted to know *why* this patient had felt no sensation of any kind while his colon was being burned. I thought this question deserved a better answer than "that is the way things are." I was confident that I could find a satisfactory answer by making a single visit to any good medical library. I think perhaps this was the first time in my life that I went eagerly to a library, not because some teacher had sent me or because I needed to cram for an examination, but because I wanted some information that I felt was important for every good surgeon to know. But I did not find the information I sought in my first session in a medical library nor in many subsequent sessions.

3

The Problem of
Visceral Sensibility

To find out why the conscious patient felt no pain while his colon was being burned, I turned first to the writings of Gaskell (1916) and Langley (1921), the authorities of that era on the functions performed by the nerves supplied to the internal organs. I had no intention of undertaking any serious study of visceral neurology. About all I knew concerning the visceral nerves was that they formed characteristic ganglia but few definite nerve trunks, and their fibers ran every which way through the mesenteries and along the walls of blood vessels to reach the internal organs. It seemed hopeless to try to trace the exact course followed by sensory fibers from the colon to the spinal cord through this fiber jungle. In fact, the whole disorderly array of visceral nerves showed so many resemblances to the nerve supply in very low forms of animal life that early investigators had considered it to be a primitive nervous system that controlled visceral function with little or no dependence on the spinal cord and brain. The investigations of Gaskell and Langley demonstrated that the visceral nerves were an integral part of the nervous system in that the control of function in all internal organs originated in the brain and spinal cord. From my point of view, this whole complex subject was a closed book that I had no desire to open. But I hoped that by skimming through the writings of these two authorities I might stumble onto a direct statement by one of them as to the presence or absence of pain fibers in the human colon.

I was disappointed to find that neither man had much to say about the sensory nerves supplied to the internal organs, as their attention was largely devoted to the two great outflow systems, sympathetic and parasympathetic, that controlled motor and secretory function in the internal organs. In 1916 Gaskell had outlined his concept of what he called the "involuntary nervous system" in these words:

> The evidence indicates that the involuntary system is built up on the same plan as the voluntary system, with receptor, connector, and excitor elements. The marked difference is that the excitor elements have left the central nervous system and become peripheral, forming the various ganglia throughout the body; while the receptor elements have remained in the same position as those of the voluntary system, namely, in the posterior root ganglia, and connect by means of sensory root fibers with cells of connector elements, which have remained within the central nervous system; the connector fibers passing out to reach their respective peripherally situated excitor elements (Gaskell 1916).

Aside from this single reference to visceral afferent neurons as having the same cell station as did somatic afferent neurons, I could find no further mention in Gaskell's writings of the contribution that sensory input from the viscera might make in the regulation of visceral functions.

Langley also devoted most of his attention to the motor outflow systems. He acknowledged the presence of sensory fibers in the internal organs and he implied that they must play an important part in the control of visceral function. But he also admitted that he did not know how their physiological properties might differ from those of somatic sensory fibers. On this point he had commented in 1903: "All that seems to me possible at present toward arranging afferent fibers into autonomic and somatic divisions, is to consider as 'afferent autonomic' those which give rise to reflexes in autonomic tissues and which are incapable of directly giving rise to sensation; and to consider all other fibers as somatic."

I interpreted this statement as meaning that if visceral afferents could "directly" give rise to sensation, Langley would assume they differed in no way from somatic afferents. Visceral afferents capable of initiating reflexes but incapable of directly giving rise to sensation presumably had different physiological properties, according to this classification. The word "directly" puzzled me. Was Langley implying that what he called "afferent autonomic" might be able to give rise to such sensation as pain in some mysterious "indirect" fashion? I did not understand this nor could I apply these statements to the colostomy problem. My patient had come to the hospital seeking relief from cramping pains in his abdomen. Both he and I had assumed they originated in his intestinal tract. If so, according to Langley, the visceral afferents giving rise to the pain must be identical with somatic afferents. Why, then, had they not behaved like somatic afferents by giving rise to pain when the colon was burned?

A quick search through other textbooks of anatomy and physiology failed to provide an answer to this question, so I turned to the writings of clinicians. I found that many surgeons had been intrigued by the same question that was troubling me and that two schools of thought had developed as to how it should be answered. According to one group, which included Lennander (1902) and MacKenzie (1909), there were *no pain fibers* supplied to internal organs. The opposing group, led by Ross (1888) and Head (1920), maintained there were pain fibers in the internal organs capable of giving rise to pain directly ascribable to the organ at fault. As I read the contributions from these two schools of thought, I found myself shifting from one interpretation to the other under the influence of their persuasive arguments.

K.G. Lennander was a German surgeon who had stoutly maintained that "all organs supplied by the sympathetic or vagus below the recurrent laryngeal have no sensation of pain, touch, heat, or cold." He had performed many surgical operations under local anesthesia and while exploring a conscious patient's belly he had carefully tested the sensitivity of each structure encountered. The parietal peritoneum proved to be exquisitely sensitive to any form of stimulation, but all the organs within the abdominal cavity seemed to be completely insensitive to mechanical, thermal, and electrical stimulation. If he avoided contact with the parietal peritoneum, the only way he could elicit a complaint of pain from his patients was to exert traction on the mesenteries attaching internal organs to the body wall. He concluded that the body wall was richly supplied with somatic pain fibers that might extend for a short distance into the mesenteries so they could be activated by traction or by inflammation in nearby lymph glands. But the internal organs apparently had no pain fibers. In some of his experiments he had stimulated the intestine with strong faradic currents, which caused the gut to blanch in strong peristaltic contractions, but at no time during such tests did the patients complain of pain. In one most drastic experiment he had distended a patient's colon with a balloon and increased the pressure until the bowel burst open, yet he stated that this patient had experienced no pain. Lennander's observations had convinced him that the only way visceral disease could produce pain was by activating somatic pain fibers in the body wall, either by mechanical stimulation or by direct extension of some inflammatory process.

At their face value, Lennander's arguments sounded convincing. I was tempted to adopt his interpretation because it would permit me to explain the colostomy incident without having to give up my push-button concept of pain. However, as I read more of what Ross, Head, and MacKenzie had said about the problem, I realized that it was not as simple as Lennander had assumed it to be. All three men were concerned with the question that was bothering me, but they seemed equally concerned with a second problem they evidently thought was related to the first. All three men seemed to be asking, "How does it happen that visceral disease often expresses itself in signs and symptoms involving somatic tissues at a distance from the diseased viscus?" The introduction of this second question initially annoyed me because I failed to see that it had any bearing on the first question. They were evidently talking about "referred pain" and I thought that I knew all it was necessary to know about this phenomenon.

For example, I would have explained the shoulder pain associated with a subphrenic abscess about like this: In early embryonic life the central portion of the diaphragm takes origin in the cervical region and derives its nerve supply from nearby cervical segments of the spinal cord. Most of its nerve fibers come to it from the fourth cervical segment and these, with small additions from the third and fifth segments, form the phrenic nerve. As the embryo grows, the diaphragm gradually moves downward to its adult situation and drags the phrenic nerve with it. When a subphrenic abscess develops, the inflammatory process irritates the sensory fibers in the phrenic nerve and the impulses they conduct centrally enter the spinal cord in close proximity to somatic sensory fibers supplied to skin over the shoulder region. Somatic tissues give rise to pain so much more easily than do visceral tissues, so any pain resulting from the diaphragm irritation is felt by the patient as originating over his shoulder.

I would have used this same facile explanation to account for the pain that is often referred to the region of the umbilicus during the onset of an acute appendicitis or the pain referred down the left arm during a bout of angina pectoris. But evidently Ross, Head, and MacKenzie were looking for a better explanation than this. None of them assumed that the visceral afferents were in direct anatomical contact with somatic afferents, but unless this assumption was made, how could nerve impulses in a visceral afferent spread to a somatic afferent?

Their individual attempts to answer this question are of more than historical interest and the similarity in their lines of reasoning is best indicated by direct quotations. As early as December 7, 1887, James Ross had read a paper before the Manchester Medical Society that was entitled, "On the Segmental Distribution of Sensory Disorders." He began this classical dissertation by attributing sensations resulting from peripheral stimulation to a "molecular disturbance" within the cells of the cerebral cortex of the brain. His chief arguments in favor of this view were: (1) If the messages from the periphery were prevented from reaching the brain by the interruption of any part of the conducting pathway, no sensation was elicited by any form of peripheral stimulation; and (2) When a "spontaneous molecular disturbance" occurs in the cortex, "as in certain cases of epilepsy," . . . "various sensations are felt at the periphery in the absence of any outward disturbance to correspond with them." Ross called attention to the segmental distribution of somatic sensory nerves and pointed out that visceral disease often expresses itself by signs and symptoms arising within these segments. He then described the characteristic pains of various visceral diseases and in each instance he tried to distinguish between what he called "splanchnic" pain (directly attributable to the organ at fault) and "somatic" pain (occurring secondarily in the segmental area of reference). For example, in a disease involving the stomach, both kinds of pain might be present; the dull ache in the epigastrium represented the splanchnic pain, while all other pains ascribed to the back, shoulders, and intercostal areas represented somatic pain. As to how the somatic pain pathways became secondarily involved, he said: "The splanchnic nerves of the stomach are derived from the fourth, fifth, and probably the sixth dorsal nerves, and when the splanchnic terminations of these nerves are irritated, the irritation is conducted to the posterior roots of the nerves and on reaching the grey matter of the posterior horns it *diffuses* into the roots of the corresponding somatic nerves and thus causes an associated pain in the territory of the distribution of these nerves, which may appropriately be named the somatic pain." (Ross 1888)

In 1893 Henry Head published the first of a series of papers in which he offered an extension of the hypothesis Ross had advanced.

This early paper was entitled "Disturbances of Sensation with Special Reference to the Pain of Visceral Disease" (Head 1893). In it appeared his first maps of the segmental areas, subsequently known as "Head's zones," in which pain, muscle spasm, and cutaneous hyperesthesia appeared in cases of herpes zoster and certain diseases of the internal organs. As to how the signs and symptoms of visceral disease might be referred to somatic segments, Head wrote:

> If the impulses pass up the nerves from an organ which is diseased, to the cord, they will set up a disturbance in the segment of the cord to which they are conducted. Now any second impulse from another part, connected to the same segment, will be profoundly affected. Under normal circumstances, it would set up its own proper disturbance, which would have been conducted to the brain. But now it no longer falls into a normal and quiescent cord, but into one whose activity is already disturbed. In many cases, the second stimulus will be exaggerated, *like rays passing through a convex glass.* Thus, if any segment of the cord is disturbed by painful stimuli from an internal organ, a stimulus applied to the skin over the areas belonging to that segment will be exaggerated and the stimulus, which normally was only uncomfortable, will now appear to be very painful.

Head agreed with Ross in thinking that, in addition to referred pain, true visceral pain existed, and this meant to him that the viscera must be supplied with intrinsic pain fibers. He based this opinion on the fact that his patients often ascribed their pain directly to the site of the diseased organ. They described such pain as coming from "deep inside" and being "dull," "heavy," and "wearing," rather than by such descriptive terms as "sharp" and "stabbing," terms that he felt were more characteristic of somatic pain.

The most distinguished representative of the school of thought which maintained that there were no pain fibers supplied to internal organs was James MacKenzie. He studied visceral pain phenomena for more than thirty years and published his first comments about it in 1893, the same year that Head recorded the interpretations quoted above. Early in MacKenzie's career, long before he became known as an authority on diseases of the heart, he had taken part in a surgical operation in which the patient's abdomen was being explored under local anesthesia. In the course of the operation a portion of the patient's intestine was observed to contract strongly at intervals, and each time it contracted the man complained of pain. He ascribed this pain to the midline, whereas the contracting loop of gut was many inches away at one side of the operative field. MacKenzie interpreted this observation as indicating that the pain was not originating in the contracting segment but was due to the secondary activation of somatic pain fibers supplied to the belly wall and referred to the midline. This interpretation was reinforced later by his studies of cases of angina pectoris in which pain was referred to the left arm. He was particularly impressed by the fact that in such cases the skin over the inner side of the left elbow sometimes remained hypersensitive for days after the acute attack had subsided. Many observations of this kind suggested to him that strong and repeated showers of afferent impulses from a diseased internal organ might create an "irritable focus" in the spinal cord gray matter that is sometimes slow in subsiding.

MacKenzie's arguments in favor of this hypothesis were remarkably similar to those used by Ross and Head to account for referred phenomena. He believed that *all* pains due to visceral disease could be accounted for by this single hypothesis and he was reluctant to adopt a second hypothesis (that true visceral pain existed) when one would do. His line of reasoning is indicated by the following quotations taken from his classical monograph *Angina Pectoris*, published in 1923. In it he said:

> When the pain that arises from a stimulus produced by an organ is felt in the neighborhood of the organ, the belief is common that the pain is felt in that organ. When, as often happens, the pain is felt at a distance from the organs and there are good grounds which show that the organ is the cause of the pain, then it is assumed that the pain does not arise directly from the organ, but by some other mechanism. If we take as our hypothesis that there is only one mechanism by which pain can be produced, then the explanation for the distribution of the pain becomes clear. Thus, there is no doubt that the pain felt in parts remote from the organ is produced by the employment of cerebrospinal nerves which supply the remote region. It is manifest, therefore, that this pain is produced by the mechanism that supplied the arm.

In speaking of the pains of angina pectoris he wrote:

> We can infer that the mechanism which produces the chest pain is the same as that which produces the arm pain, and investigation by appropriate methods leaves little doubt as to this being true. Thus, a patient may have pain starting in the chest, and as it increases in severity it gradually

extends from the centre of the chest outward to the axilla and down the left arm. It is reasonable to infer that the pain of the arm is but an extension of that felt in the chest and that the mechanism is the same in both cases. This view is strengthened by the fact that in some patients the pain may be first in the arm and as it gradually increases in severity it may extend up the arm and settle in the chest.

The more I read of the interpretations of these three famous clinicians the more excited I became. I felt that I was learning something of great importance, although I was not sure what there was about the information that made it important to know. Although these men were advancing hypotheses that had no supporting experimental evidence, all three evidently had a much more dynamic concept of pain than I had learned. They were assuming that afferent impulses from a diseased organ were capable of setting up some kind of abnormal activity involving nerve cells in a segment of the spinal cord. Ross had thought that this "irritation" could "diffuse" into somatic sensory neurons to cause pain. Head thought the "disturbance of function" could exaggerate the sensory input by some focusing process, "like rays passing through a convex glass," while MacKenzie had labeled the segmental disturbance an "irritable focus" because its effect on the somatic input might outlast the visceral input.

Exciting as these new ideas were at the time, I could not see that they solved the problems created by the colostomy incident, nor did I know how I might incorporate these ideas into my push-button concept of pain. But I began an eager search for referred phenomena in every case of visceral disease I encountered, and whenever I took part in an operation performed under local anesthesia I made tentative tests of visceral sensibility. Although their scope was limited, all the observations that I made during these two years of surgical training served to increase my interest in the problem of visceral pain. I found myself increasingly favoring MacKenzie's interpretation of referred phenomena and willing to believe that there were no specific pain fibers supplied to the internal organs. At least, if there were any pain fibers in the viscera their physiological properties must be quite different from those of the somatic pain fibers. Perhaps one reason I tended to favor MacKenzie's theory was that it did least damage to my original concept of pain. However, I found it difficult to believe that in colostomy patients cramping pains could be adequately accounted for by postulating the existence of an irritable focus in the spinal cord.

4

The Adequate Stimulus
For True Visceral Pain

After I established an office in Portland it was a long time before I had many private patients to care for, so I spent most of my time in the library and clinics of the University of Oregon Medical School. I joined the surgical staff and was given permission to carry on my study of pain in both the laboratory and the hospital. I was even permitted to offer two elective courses of lectures to medical students in their junior and senior years. The lectures offered to junior students dealt with "Visceral Pain" and those offered to seniors dealt with "The Surgery of the Sympathetic Nervous System." The number of students in these classes was never large, so discussion of pain problems was always free and informal and I think I learned as much from the students as they did from me.

At first I stuck closely to the orthodox teachings about pain, except that I invoked MacKenzie's hypothesis, which assumed that visceral disease could only give rise to pain by setting up some disturbance of function in segments of the spinal cord that could secondarily activate somatic pain pathways. However, I had great difficulty convincing students that colic did not arise directly from contractions of the intestine. One of them called my attention to the 1911 Goulstonian lecture by Arthur Hurst in which he had claimed that abnormal degrees of tension acting on the walls of any hollow viscus was an "adequate" stimulus for true visceral pain. Hurst and his co-workers had put balloons into the esophagus and stomach of human subjects and had demonstrated that distention of these structures gave rise to pain that was promptly relieved when the intramural pressure was reduced (Hurst 1911). The stu-

25

dent who called attention to these experiments said he would bet that MacKenzie wouldn't have been able to refute Hurst's arguments. I knew that MacKenzie had known about Hurst's experiments but had not believed that they conclusively proved that the pain originated directly in the wall of the distended viscus. He had pointed out that in these experiments the test subjects had always ascribed pain to the midline and, although the site of the balloon might have been close to the midline, the pain might well have been somatic in origin and referred to the midline. In support of this conviction he had told Hurst about his observation of the case in which contractions of the intestinal loop situated far from the midline had given rise to pain ascribed to the midline.

Then, late in 1925, I developed a kidney infection and sought treatment by a urologist. In the course of his investigations he catheterized my ureters and filled each kidney pelvis with a dilute sodium iodide solution to visualize these structures in an X-ray picture. As he was injecting the fluid into one kidney pelvis I experienced a deep, aching pain that seemed to originate from about where I assumed the left kidney must lie. I asked him which kidney pelvis he was injecting, and when he told me it was the left one I asked him to inject the fluid two more times and to use more pressure each time so I could be a little more sure just where the pain seemed to arise. The second injection gave rise to quite a severe pain, which I felt sure must be originating in the kidney itself and to have nothing to do with the superficial tissues. I have no way of estimating the pressure he used in making the third injection, but it felt to me that the kidney had burst and I suddenly and unexpectedly vomited all over myself and his examining table. It was a most unpleasant experience that I would not care to repeat and it left me with a permanent aversion for any instrumental invasions of my body orifices. But it did serve to convince me, as no amount of argument could have done, that true visceral pain was a reality.

After this experience it seemed necessary to undertake a few experiments of my own in the hope of straightening out my concept of pain before presuming to pass it on to medical students. Now that I was convinced that internal organs were supplied with pain fibers, I ought to try to determine in what ways they differed functionally from somatic pain fibers because it was obvious that they behaved differently in response to certain noxious stimuli. Apparently visceral pain fibers could be activated by only a few of the noxious stimuli that could activate somatic pain fibers, but which ones were they? One other hypothesis ought to be tested and it had to do with the density of the population of pain fibers in skin and viscera. Perhaps visceral afferents would behave like somatic afferents if a sufficient number of them could be activated simultaneously. Between 1925 and 1928, when I left to serve a residency in surgery at Lakeside Hospital in Cleveland, I conducted a long series of tests of visceral sensibility on myself and on patients in the Multnomah County Hospital. I repeated most of the tests previously reported by other investigators and added a few modifications of my own.

Most of my experiments were carried out on patients with open colostomies who were willing to let me blindfold them while they were reporting the subjective experiences I could elicit by stimulating the exposed loop of colon. No chemical that I applied to such a loop gave rise to any sensation. Among the chemical substances I used were strong acids and alkalis, ethers and alcohols, oil of cloves and chloral hydrate. None elicited the slightest sensation of touch, heat, cold, or pain, either at the time of application or subsequently. This was true no matter how corrosive the chemical might be or the size of the area of application. Nor did any form of mechanical stimulation elicit any sensory response if I was careful not to stimulate the surrounding skin. Crushing a huge area of colon wall in a forceps was not felt nor did cutting or pricking either the serosa or the mucosa elicit any sensation. To test the "density hypothesis" I used both pricking and heat stimulations. In the first type of test I used a flat piece of hard rubber through which I had thrust fifty sharp needles. Pressing this "hair-brush" of needles against the loop failed to elicit any sensation if no pressure was transmitted to the skin. To test the response to burning, I used a flat piece of iron, about three inches long and an inch wide, which I could hold in a long, curved forceps while heating. The iron strip could be laid flat against the loop of the exposed gut, but it made no difference whether it was merely warm or red-hot; the test subject felt no pain.

There were only two ways in which I could elicit a pain response from any of these colostomy patients and I will describe these methods in relation to my favorite collaborator. "Charlotte Brown" was a charming little old lady of 72 who had an inoperable cancer of her lower bowel and whose colostomy loop was unusually redundant. She was not only a good test subject because of the size of the loop, but in addition she was an exceptionally intelligent woman who was delighted to take part in the experiments. Every time I came to visit her, carrying my testing paraphernalia, she would greet me eagerly, tie on her blindfold, and announce that she was all ready to start any tests I might suggest. The easiest way to elicit a complaint of pain from Mrs. Brown was to distend some part of her colon with a balloon. For this purpose I used a rubber condom tied over a fairly rigid catheter and connected to a Sorenson insufflator, an instrument ordinarily used to inflate fallopian tubes with oxygen under controlled pressures. When the balloon was in the colon, either proximally or distally, and it was distended at approximately 80 mm Hg pressure, Mrs. Brown reported feeling an aching pain that she ascribed to the lower part of her abdomen. It was hard for her to localize the pain exactly but it seemed to be in the midline between her umbilicus and the pubis. If the pressure was increased above this level and maintained for any length of time she said she felt as if something inside the abdomen was about to burst. She did not think she had ever before experienced a pain exactly like it but she thought it was something like the sensation she had felt when her bladder was painfully distended. However, she was certain that the pain did not originate in her bladder, although she tended to rub her hand over the bladder region when the pain was most intense. She never localized the pain very near the actual location of the balloon, as far as I could tell, a fact that might suggest that the pain was "referred" and hence of somatic rather than visceral origin. Against this interpretation was the fact that she was sure the pain did not originate in the belly wall. She said it was always "deep down, inside" and she was convinced that the pain originated in her colon. The pain, no matter how severe, was always promptly relieved as soon as the intramural pressure dropped below 80 mm Hg pressure.

Mrs. Brown reported quite a different kind of pain when the colon loop contracted strongly under electrical stimulation by a large inductorium. She felt nothing when the current was first applied nor when the gut first began to contract and change color. As the peristaltic contraction blanched the loop she complained of a gradually increasing pain, which she said was like a "gas pain." If the gut contracted strongly enough to lose almost all of its pink color, the pain became quite severe and she compared it with a "green apple colic." She described the wave-like character of the pain: a gradual ascent, a plateau, and then a gradual fading as the gut relaxed. I noted that the pain had entirely disappeared before the gut had regained its normal red color and long after the stimulating electrodes had been withdrawn. Of course, during these tests she could hear the buzzing of the inductorium, yet neither this wound nor any leading questions I might ask could influence her to make false reports of her sensory experiences.

A few months after completing these tests on Charlotte Brown, I was called to see a patient whose history indicated that she had suffered from both kinds of visceral pain. She was a Christian Science practitioner of 52 who had been suffering from a complete intestinal obstruction for seven days. She was in critical condition due to dehydration and exhaustion and her abdomen was enormously distended and as tight and tympanic as a drum. One puzzling feature of her story was that her attendants had given her many enemas but in each instance, although the water had run in quite freely, almost none of it came back. I could feel nothing in her rectum; the tightness and tenderness of the belly wall made it impossible to feel anything through it. She was taken at once to the hospital where an X-ray picture showed both the small and large intestines to be greatly distended and arranged in a ladder-like series of horizontal layers of fluid and gas, the typical picture of an acute intestinal obstruction low down in the colon. An operation showed the cause of the obstruction to be an exceptionally large gallstone at the end of the sigmoid flexure. This gallstone had evidently eroded through the wall of the gallbladder into the transverse colon and then had passed down to lodge at the brim of the pelvis, where it had acted like a ball-valve when the patient was given enemas.

The main point of interest in this case was her story of pain. For the first three or four days of her illness she had suffered from intermittent cramping pains that steadily increased in violence and frequency. Associated with these pains was an expulsive type of vomiting of clear fluid, tinged with bile. By the end of the fourth day her abdomen was greatly distended and her vomiting changed from its previous explosive violence to a passive regurgitation of fecal smelling, brownish fluid. At the same time her pain changed from cramping to a steady ache that seemed to involve the entire abdomen. By the sixth day the pain had become almost unbearable and was described as a "bursting" sensation that was little affected by the analgesic drugs her attendants administered hypodermically. By the seventh day the woman was so exhausted she could no longer tolerate her pain and both she and her attendants momentarily expected that her abdomen might burst open. It was only then that she consented to have a surgeon called in to treat her.

The recent observations I had made as to the possible causes for visceral pain helped me reconstruct the chain of events that must have been taking place within this patient's abdomen. The early cramping pains were obviously caused by the violent peristaltic contractions of the intestine in its efforts to force its fluid content past the obstructing gallstones. The pains were wave-like in character and typical of what is often called "muscle spasm." When the peristaltic contractions failed to expel the fluid content, waves of reversed peristalsis brought on the expulsive vomiting of bile-tinged fluid. As the patient's condition deteriorated and the distention of the gut stretched the smooth muscle beyond its power to contract, the explosive vomiting was replaced by a passive regurgitation of fluid contaminated with lower bowel content. At this time the second type of pain developed and the cramping pains were replaced by a continuous ache that made her think something inside the belly was about to burst open. Finally, as the viability of the intestinal wall became impaired, fluid began to leak out into the belly cavity and a third type of pain was added. This could be attributed to irritation of the sensitive parietal peritoneum and as the general peritonitis developed, muscle spasm, tenderness to pressure, and pain of somatic origin added to the clinical picture.

5

"Visceral Pain" from Peripheral Blood Vessels

In the early years of my private practice I had among my patients a number of men and women seeking treatment for troublesome varicosities in their leg veins. I operated on some of these patients by using the method of treatment I had learned during my hospital internship, that of stripping out long segments of disabled veins on a metal "stripper." This form of treatment gave satisfactory results, but a new ambulatory treatment was coming into vogue and patients were beginning to ask for it because it could be given in a series of treatments instead of requiring an operation and a stay in the hospital. In this new treatment the veins were injected with a sclerosing solution that caused a thrombus to form inside the vein; the solution caused an inflammation of the vein wall sufficient to firmly anchor the thrombus. I tried this method of treatment on a few patients by using a sclerosing agent that was a mixture of equal parts of 50% glucose solution and 20% salt solution. This solution was heavy and viscid and required a large needle because of the need to use great care during the injection to avoid leakage outside the vein. Any escape of this fluid outside the vein set up an intense inflammation of the tissues, which sometimes broke down to form an ulcer that was slow to heal. Even when there was no leakage around the needle, patients often complained of a severe cramping pain in the lower leg after the completion of the injection. In the medical literature this cramping pain was referred to as a "muscle ache," and I assumed that it originated in the leg muscles until a frightening experience convinced me that the pain originated in the vein wall.

One day a dermatologist from a neighboring office asked me to examine a patient of his and give my advice as to whether he needed an injection in one of his leg veins. I was told that this patient was a rich lumberman of the "high-pressure-executive type" whom the dermatologist had been treating for some time in an effort to clear up a "pellagra-like" skin eruption on his forearms and lower legs. No form of treatment seemed to have any effect on the skin eruption and the patient was becoming highly vocal in his criticisms. With the hope of uncovering some systemic cause for the skin condition, the dermatologist had sent the patient to an internist for a searching examination. The internist found nothing wrong with the man that might be related to his skin condition. However, during his examination he did notice a moderate enlargement of the patient's internal saphenous vein and he had commented at the time that if this vein increased in size and began to cause symptoms it might be advisable to have it injected. He assured the patient that this symptomless vein enlargement had nothing to do with the skin eruption, but now that this patient was back in the dermatologist's office he was demanding to have the vein injected. He told the dermatologist that there was no sense in waiting until this vein caused trouble and he wanted it injected "right now."

I found the vein to be moderately enlarged but it showed no true varicosities and I told the patient I saw no need to inject it because it was causing no symptoms and had no possible relation to his skin eruption. However, the patient demanded immediate injection and the dermatologist urged me to do it, evidently glad to get this patient off his back for a time. I reluctantly took the patient back to my office and prepared to give him an injection. While I was drawing the sclerosing solution into the syringe, he sat on my examining table asking a lot of questions about the procedure: how painful it was, would it lay him up, how many injections would be necessary, etc., etc. He urged me to give him a big injection because he had no intention of "hanging around for a lot of fool injections." It was my usual custom, in starting a series of injections for a new patient, to begin with a small one and then gauge the amount to be used in subsequent injections by the reaction it produced. This time, however, I was foolish enough to be influenced by this man's demands for a large injection and drew into the syringe the full 10 cc of the solution, which I considered to be the "maximal" dose.

With the patient standing, the needle was introduced into the lumen of the vein a short distance below his knee. I injected all of the solution, withdrew the needle, and applied pressure over the puncture site. While pressing on this spot I happened to notice that the enlarged vein was disappearing down near his ankle. As I watched this interesting phenomenon, the patient groaned loudly and began to sway. I looked up to see that he was ghastly pale, and I just managed to break his fall as he slumped to the office floor. He was deeply unconscious and inert as I lifted him onto the examination table. His hands and face were white and wet with sweat. His pulse was so rapid and thready that I had trouble finding it. I feared that he was dying. I elevated the foot of the table and was wondering what I had best do next when the color began to return to his face and he gave signs of recovering consciousness. When he was fully conscious, he told me he had felt nothing unpleasant beyond the needle prick until after the solution had all been injected and the needle withdrawn. He had just decided that "there is nothing to it" when he experienced a "horrible cramp" near his ankle, "as if the ankle was being crushed in a vise." This pain seemed to get worse as it ascended the leg and he felt "lightheaded." He could remember having groaned but did not know that he had fallen.

I kept this man under observation in my office for the rest of the afternoon. When his wife arrived to take him home I asked him to report immediately by phone if he had any recurrence of symptoms; otherwise he was to return in a week. He did not keep this appointment. I let another week go and then called the dermatologist. "Yes," he had heard from the lumberman by phone to the effect that my treatment had almost killed him and damned if he would visit my office again. A few weeks later the dermatologist called me in great excitement to say that the patient was in his office and I must come in to see the remarkable change in his condition. He had not examined the man's leg, but the amazing thing was that the skin eruption had disappeared. When I entered the other office it was apparent that the patient was better disposed toward me, evidently thinking that drastic treatment had cured his skin condition.

Neither the dermatologist nor I could account for the sudden disappearance of the skin eruption. We thought that if this was more than a coincidence, the change must have been due to the profound shock to this man's system produced by the pain rather than to the injection itself. The saphenous vein was no longer visible but along its course I could palpate a thin, hard cord about the size of a telephone wire, extending from the inner side of his ankle to his groin. As I tried to reconstruct what might have happened, I decided that the heavy solution had drifted rapidly down inside the vein to the ankle level where it had caused so much irritation that the smooth muscle in the vein wall went into spasm. This tended to squeeze the solution upward in the vein in sufficient concentration to produce more irritation and muscle spasm until the entire internal saphenous vein was involved. I judged that the muscular contraction in this relatively normal vein was so intense that a barrage of afferent impulses had poured into his central nervous system to induce a state of shock. As the shock and pain increased, a drop in blood pressure had caused him to lose consciousness and fall.

Fortunately, I never again had a patient complain of a "muscle ache" as severe as this man had experienced, nor did I ever again ascribe these pains to the skeletal muscle. I felt confident that the pain had originated in the vein wall and was due to spasm of the relatively intact smooth muscle. To confirm this conviction, I began keeping a careful record of every kind of pain reported by my patients either during or after the vein injections. These records suggested that four different kinds of pain were distinguishable, two that I believed were somatic in origin and two that I called visceral because they resembled the two kinds of pain that can be elicited experimentally from the intestine.

The first of the pains I called somatic was a burning, smarting, sensation coming on while the injection was in progress. I attributed it to the irritant effect of the sclerosing solution on perivascular tissues due to small amounts of the solution on the needle or leaking back from the venipuncture. The second somatic pain came on a few days after the injection had been given, at a time when the inflammatory reaction inside the vein was at its height. I attributed this pain to an extension of the inflammation into tissues around the vein and I noticed that it was most apt to appear while the patient was walking or touching the area around the inflamed vein.

The first of the pains I called visceral was described as a dull, deep ache that appeared whenever an isolated segment of vein was distended with fluid. This ache appeared whether the distention was produced by the sclerosing solution or by an injection of normal salt solution, and it disappeared promptly when the intramural tension was reduced by drawing some of the fluid back into the syringe. The second visceral pain was the type described in the medical literature as a "deep muscle ache." In its milder forms this pain was described as a deep cramp and when it was severe as "vise-like" or "crushing." It usually started after the injection was completed and the needle had been withdrawn, approximately seventy seconds after the solution first began entering the vein. For about forty-five seconds the pain gradually increased; it remained severe for another minute and then faded slowly. If the vein was relatively normal as in the lumberman's case, the cramping pain might last somewhat longer but it was usually all done within three to five minutes.

The idea that visceral pain might originate in peripheral blood vessels was new to me at the time I began making these observations, but I found that many other clinicians had reached the same conclusion on the basis of experimental observations. Odermatt (1922) had reported some animal experiments that had convinced him that pain originated in the walls of both arteries and veins, either when they were being distended under high pressure or were contracting strongly when irritated by the injection of chemicals within their lumina. He attributed pain due to distention to the stretching of perivascular sensory endings he called "visceral afferent neurons." When he injected barium chloride into a dog's brachial artery the animal showed unmistakable signs of severe pain, which Odermatt thought was due to smooth muscle spasm, and he believed this type of pain was exactly similar to the pain of intestinal colic.

One of the first clinicians to ascribe visceral pain to peripheral blood vessels was René Leriche of Strasbourg. His pioneer studies of causalgia, phantom limb pain, and other bizarre pain states had convinced him as early as 1913 that what he called "sympathetic pain" could arise from all visceral structures, either from internal organs or from the smooth muscle in the peripheral blood vessels (Leriche 1913). He maintained that this pain is altogether different from the pains due to any form of noxious stimulation applied to somatic tissues. He ascribed "sympathetic pain" to irritation of visceral afferents in the walls of blood vessels and he assumed that these fibers followed along the walls for considerable distances and eventually reached the spinal cord by way of the chain of sympathetic ganglia within the body cavities. In support of this interpretation he cited the extraordinary success he had had in relieving sympathetic pain by excising appropriate sympathetic ganglia or by doing a "periarterial sympathectomy," which consisted of stripping off the adventitia of the main artery proximal to the source of the pain.

However, experimental studies on animals in the laboratories of anatomists and physiologists had failed to support Leriche's interpretations. For example, the investigations of Kramer and Todd (1914) had indicated that no sensory fibers traveled for any considerable distance along the walls of the blood vessels. Instead, the evidence indicated that they promptly entered spinal nerve trunks and entered the spinal cord by way of the posterior root ganglia and did *not* traverse sympathetic ganglia. All I had read by 1930 uncovered no experimental evidence to support Leriche's contentions, and the consensus among physiologists could be summarized in these three statements:

1. The sensory fibers supplied to peripheral blood vessels differ in no essential features from somatic afferents. They have exactly the same anatomical distribution and apparently possess the same physiological properties.

2. No rational explanation can be offered to account for the relief of pain that has been ascribed to either a periarterial sympathectomy or to a ganglionectomy.

3. A sympathetic ganglionectomy produces a transient vasodilation but this temporary improvement in the peripheral blood supply to the part disappears as soon as the postganglionic fiber degenerates. The blood vessels are thereafter hypersensitive to the vasoconstrictive effect of circulating adrenaline.

These conclusions, based on animal experimentation, tended to discredit Leriche's interpretations and raised questions as to the reliability of his observations and the reported results of his surgical operations. I felt that these implied criticisms of Leriche's contributions were unfair. He may well have been wrong in his assumptions as to the route by which visceral afferents reached the spinal cord, but the results of his operations were astonishingly good. Based on my limited experience in this field, I felt there was no good reason to question Leriche's claims. At least, I was certain that the physiologists were wrong in asserting that a sympathectomy never produced more than a transient vasodilation in human patients. Before I explain the basis for this opinion, a brief sketch of the history of the operation called a "sympathec-tomy" is in order.

In 1851 Claude Bernard published the results of some experiments on animals showing that the cutting of sympathetic nerves supplied to an extremity was followed by a marked dilatation of the peripheral blood vessels and an increase in the temperature of the affected limb (Bernard 1851). He assumed that he had severed "motor" fibers supply-ing the smooth muscle of blood vessels but noted that the smooth muscle neither exhibited a flaccid paralysis nor subsequently degener-ated, as was true for skeletal muscle after its motor supply has been divided. Bernard recorded the fact, later to be confirmed by physiolo-gists, that in experimental animals the period of vasodilation disap-peared within two or three weeks after the sympathectomy and the vessels resumed their previous caliber. Weir Mitchell was a pupil of Bernard's about this time and may well have taken part in these pio-neer studies of vasomotor control. In any event, Mitchell repeated these same experiments in 1871 in an effort to throw some light on the vasomotor disturbances he had observed as a characteristic feature of the terrible pain syndrome he named causalgia. However, Mitchell's animal experiments did little to help him explain causalgia because they merely confirmed Bernard's finding of a transient vasodilation, whereas the vasomotor disturbances in causalgia persisted for months or years.

As far as I can determine, the first surgeon to excise sympathetic ganglia in a human patient in the hope of augmenting the peripheral circulation was William Alexander of Liverpool. In 1889 he published a book reporting his experiences with cervical ganglionectomy to treat epilepsy (Alexander 1889). Although the results he obtained were not encouraging, other surgeons subsequently performed sympathectomies for a variety of apparently unrelated conditions such as exophthalmic goiter, idiocy, and asthma. However, it was soon evident that the pro-cedure conferred no lasting benefit in these conditions. In 1889 Jaboulay of Lyon reported that he had brought about healing in an indolent, "penetrating," and painful ulcer on a man's foot by stripping off the outer coat of the femoral artery of the affected limb. In 1915 Leriche tried this same arterial stripping on a soldier who had sustained a bullet wound through his right axilla five days previously (Leriche 1916). This man had complained of a terrible burning pain in the right arm and hand, the clinical picture being similar to the syndrome Mitchell had called "causalgia." Leriche thought that the coldness, cyanosis, and excessive sweating in this soldier's arm and hand indicated an overactivity in the sympathetic nerve supply, and this first "periarterial sympathectomy" was undertaken to remove the sympathetic influence on the vessels of the limb. This operation greatly reduced the patient's pain and improved the peripheral circulation. However, a complete cure of the condition was not established until after Leriche had found and excised a thrombosed segment of the axillary artery near the site of the bullet wound. From that time on, Leriche conceived of causalgia as representing a "wound of the sympathetic" and he became an ardent advocate of arterial stripping, arterectomy, ganglionectomy, and ramicotomy for the treatment of any chronic pain state in which there was any evidence of a persistent disturbance of function in peripheral blood vessels.

Jonnesco (1920) reported that he had been successful in ridding a patient of severe bouts of angina pectoris by removing the stellate and inferior cervical ganglia on the left side of this patient's neck. Jonnesco reported that the anginal attacks had stopped immediately after the sympathectomy and had not recurred during the two years he had kept this patient under observation. Other surgeons began to do sympathectomies for the relief of anginal pain, and though the location and extent of their excisions varied widely, they all reported good results in some of their patients. Royle, an Australian surgeon, recommended sympathectomy for the relief of spastic paralysis in children (Royle 1927). During wide travels in the United States, Royle showed pictures of the cases he had operated on and reported the improvement they exhibited after an appropriate ganglionectomy. Adson and Craig of the Mayo Clinic performed Royle's operation and they were greatly impressed by the marked improvement that the procedure effected in the blood flow in the legs and feet of these patients. After the operation the feet became warm, pink, and dry and calorimetric studies indicated that the local heat production had increased by two to nine times its previous level. Still more interesting was the fact that the circulatory improvement persisted rather than faded within three weeks, as experiments on animals had led them to expect. Adson and Craig then began doing sympathectomies on patients suffering from various kinds of peripheral vascular disturbance (Craig 1931; Adison 1930).

In 1930 Adson and Rowntree reported a few cases of chronic arthritis that had apparently benefited from operations on appropriate parts of the sympathetic chain of ganglia. They said the immediate improvement in blood flow in the affected limb had relieved much of the pain and disability in these cases and they suggested the possibility that the improvement in tissue nutrition might eventually reverse the underlying pathological changes in the bones and joints. In discussing their arthritic patients, they wrote: "The patients we have selected for operation are those who complained of painful swollen joints, associated with limited motion, atrophy of muscles, and loss of function, and who also complained of cold extremities, mild acrocyanosis, excessive perspiration, and aggravated symptoms during stormy weather. One of our patients described her feet and legs by saying they felt like dead fish, thus effectively describing the cold, clammy skin of the extremities."

The wave of enthusiasm that swept the country following the publication of this report died out as soon as it became clear that a sympathectomy cannot "cure" any type of arthritis, and this disease was added to the long list of clinical syndromes that sympathectomies had failed to benefit. Nevertheless, this surgical adventure was one of the landmarks in the progress of visceral nerve surgery. Nothing that had gone before had done so much to arouse the interest of surgeons and physiologists in the study of visceral nerve functions. The trouble was that conclusions based on animal experiments, as I have listed them previously, seemed to show that a sympathectomy could produce no more than a transient improvement in the peripheral blood supply to a limb and that visceral afferents do *not* traverse the sympathetic ganglia to reach the spinal cord. Why, then, did surgeons persist in their claims that a sympathectomy could alleviate certain chronic pain states and bring about a lasting increase in the peripheral blood flow? If surgeons of that era had attempted to answer this question, I would have joined them in saying, "We do not know just how a sympathectomy produces these favorable effects but the fact is, it can and does produce them in well-selected cases."

6

Studies of Visceral Nerve Function

W hile serving a surgical residency in Lakeside Hospital in Cleveland, I performed my first Jonnesco type of sympath-ectomy on a patient suffering from frequent and severe bouts of anginal pain. The operation was successful in relieving the man's pain and greatly increased his exercise tolerance. Because of this good result and knowing of my interest in all problems of visceral nerve function, Elliott Cutler, my chief of surgery, permitted me to do a number of sympathectomies during my residency period. Prior to that time I had done one or two periarterial sympathectomies and a few ganglionectomies. But the few I had done had convinced me that ex-periments on normal laboratory animals were not an adequate basis for predicting the results of sympathectomy on human patients suffering from vasomotor disturbances. Most of the cases I had operated on had been subjected to skin temperature studies prior to operation to deter-mine the degree of vasospasm present in each case. In my hands, this prognostic test was more reliable than either the "fever test" or oscillo-metric studies. Whenever a procaine block of the appropriate sympa-thetic ganglia was followed immediately by a striking rise in skin tem-perature, I felt confident that a ganglionectomy would be followed by an increase in the peripheral circulation that would persist indefinitely.

I remember showing George Burget, our professor of physiology, one of the cases in which I had done a right lumbar sympathectomy five years previously. This woman's right foot had remained warm and dry and she said she used it as she would a hotwater bottle with which to warm her cold, damp left foot when she went to bed each night.

I asked George why he thought the results of the sympathectomy in this case differed so strikingly from the results of the same operation on laboratory animals. We decided that the most likely answer to this question must be "because normal animals do not suffer from the same vasomotor disturbances that cause pain and disability in human patients." Our reasoning went about like this: If it could be shown that a patient's peripheral blood vessels were constantly subject to abnormal degrees of constriction, we would expect that a sympathectomy would remove this vasoconstrictive influence. The vessels would then exhibit the same transient vasodilation that they showed in normal animals subjected to the same procedure. As soon as the postganglionic fibers had degenerated, the peripheral vessels would resume a "normal" degree of tonus, exactly as had been demonstrated for laboratory animals. Moreover, the human blood vessels might then be abnormally sensitive to the effects of circulating adrenaline. However, once the patient's blood vessels had been released from the vasoconstrictor influence of the sympathetic fibers, the caliber of the vessels in a state of "normal" tonus might be much greater than it had been prior to operation.

Once we had admitted that the physiologists might not have been on solid ground in saying that a sympathectomy could never induce a persistent increase in the peripheral circulation, we began to wonder if they might not have been wrong in denying that visceral afferents from blood vessels reached the spinal cord by way of the sympathetic chain of ganglia. In performing their experiments, perhaps the physiologists had failed to elicit true visceral pain—that is, pain actually arising in the walls of arteries or veins. We might be able to test this hypothesis by cutting all the posterior roots in a dog's brachial plexus and then injecting some highly irritant chemical into its brachial artery. If the injection produced immediate and unmistakable evidences of pain we could conclude that the sensation reached the central nervous system by some less direct route, perhaps by way of the gray rami and the ganglionic chain. Further testing of this hypothesis might be obtained by excising portions of the chain of ganglia to see if the removal altered the evidences of pain. During 1930 we carried out a series of experiments according to this general design. Our observations were published in the May 1931 issue of the *American Journal of Physiology* (Burget 1931) and our conclusions read as follows:

1. Injection of 5% lactic acid into the brachial artery of a dog gives rise to afferent impulses which apparently are painful to the animals.

2. This reaction is dependent upon changes in the vessel wall rather than on secondary changes in somatic tissues.

3. The removal of stellate and second thoracic ganglia on one side does not alter the responses of the animal to injections of lactic acid into the brachial artery of that side.

4. These afferent impulses enter the spinal cord largely by way of the posterior roots of the seventh, eighth, and first dorsal nerves.

Thus our findings agreed with those previously reported by physiologists. Whatever a sympathectomy might have to do with pain arising from peripheral blood vessels, the benefit conferred by this operation apparently could not be ascribed to the severance of a pain pathway.

I learned a great deal in the months that I worked with George in his physiology laboratory. Part of what I learned had to do with investigative techniques, but I learned even more by watching the progress of two other investigations being carried out by other men in the same laboratory. I wish to describe these investigations because they changed my concept of how the central nervous system may function. In the first of these studies, John Clelland was trying to identify the posterior roots by which sensory fibers from a dog's uterus entered the spinal cord. In a preliminary study he had demonstrated that when the uterus is distended with fluid under considerable pressure, both rectus muscles in the abdominal wall contract strongly. As he reported later in a published paper, "A sudden increase in the intrauterine pressure to 100 mm of Hg was the minimal 'adequate' stimulus to produce a contraction of both rectus muscles, simultaneously." By using pressures above this minimum level he could record the contractions of these muscles on a kymograph. Such a recording could then be used as an indicator of sensory nerve activation, after which he could successively divide the posterior roots of the dog's spinal cord until the reflex disappeared. In this way he could map out the full extent of the sensory nerve supply to the uterus.

Clelland had tested a sufficient number of female dogs to be confident that as long as any sensory fibers from the uterus were intact, any rise of intrauterine pressure above the threshold level would elicit the reflex response. But one day he encountered an experimental animal whose rectus muscles did not respond to uterine distention in the usual fashion. Instead of contracting when the pressure in the uterus rose, the rectus muscles relaxed. He subsequently described this as "the graph of an inverted visceromotor response." This unusual reflex response puzzled him and he called George and me to observe it and help him explain it. We finally discovered that this particular dog was in an early stage of pregnancy, a fact that had escaped his notice when he had set up the experiment. Subsequent tests on other pregnant dogs confirmed that during pregnancy and for some four weeks postpartum, the rectus muscles tended to relax, rather than to contract, when the uterus was distended under pressure.

To explain this remarkable reversal of the usual reflex response we found it necessary to invoke a teleologic explanation. We assumed that it would be in the best interests of a nonpregnant female to extrude any foreign body that might invade her uterus. Nature had apparently provided her with a protective mechanism that was triggered by any sudden rise in intrauterine pressure and that would elicit expulsive efforts by the abdominal muscles and in the uterine musculature. Evidently the strong contractions of the rectus muscles that Clelland had been recording in his previous experiments were an important part of this protective mechanism. We assumed further that during pregnancy this type of reflex response would have to be suppressed if the fetus was to be permitted to grow in a normal fashion. Indeed, the reflex would have to be reversed so that the rectus muscle would progressively relax to give the expanding uterus plenty of room in the belly cavity.

Teleological explanations are always open to question, but we were unable to account for Clelland's observation otherwise. I had great difficulty in accepting it, not because I have any real objections to teleological explanations but because it didn't jibe with my concept of a reflex. I had always thought of a reflex in terms of the diagram of a "simple reflex arc." It shows one sensory neuron carrying impulses into the spinal cord and a single motor neuron to elicit the appropriate response in skeletal muscle. When I had watched Clelland's experiments and seen the rectus muscles contract each time the uterus was expanded, it had seemed to me that this response was as simple and direct as a knee jerk. How could pregnancy reverse this response? Could it be that a change in the body's internal secretions had the power to suppress a built-in neural mechanism and replace it with another better adapted to it needs? I did not know how to answer such questions but my concept of neural mechanisms was certainly being loosened up.

In the second interesting investigation being conducted in the physiology laboratory at that time, Karl Martsloff was studying acute intestinal obstruction. In those days many surgeons believed that an essential part of every operation for acute obstruction was to drain off all the retained secretion in the distended intestinal loops above the obstruction. They thought it was the "toxicity" of these retained fluids that caused the nausea, vomiting, and prostration that made the individual so terribly ill when the intestinal tract was obstructed. One of the objectives of the investigation I am about to describe was to test this assumption. For this purpose, dogs with a closed intestinal loop were used. To prepare such an animal, the investigator isolated from the rest of the intestinal tract a loop of ileum with a good blood supply and sewed its proximal and distal ends together to form a closed loop. Then, the cut ends of the small intestine were joined to restore continuity of the intestinal tract. When the operative wound was being repaired the isolated loop was fixed in position immediately below the line of suture so that when the wound had healed the loop would lie directly beneath the midpoint of the belly scar. Such an animal would then have an unobstructed intestinal tract for the passage of food products but the contents of the closed loop could not escape unless the experimenters drew it off with a needle. This could be done by plunging a needle through the operative scar into the lumen of the closed loop in much the same way as one can pump up or let down the air pressure in a basketball by inserting a needle through a special plug of soft rubber in the ball's surface. In this way, the investigators could draw off fluids secreted within the loop and could either raise or lower the pressure inside the loop.

With this experimental setup a dog never developed any of the signs and symptoms of intestinal obstruction as long as the pressure within the closed loop was kept at a low level. It seemed to make no difference in the dog's condition whether the fluid allowed to remain within the loop was retained secretion with its decomposition products or normal salt solution. As long as the loop was prevented from becoming distended, the dog ate well, was playful and was apparently normal in all its behavior. Yet if the pressure within the loop was raised above 80 mm Hg, the dog became ill. The first sign was that the animal became restless and refused both food and water. When a pan of fresh meat was placed before him he would turn away from it as if in disgust. If the pressure within the loop was not promptly reduced, the dog would begin to retch and vomit and become progressively dehydrated and prostrated. Left untreated, the dog would eventually die after showing all of the signs and symptoms of human patients when their intestinal tract is completely obstructed. However, if this chain of events is not allowed to progress too far, it is promptly terminated as soon as the pressure within the loop has dropped below the critical level.

I was particularly interested in the behavior of the dogs who had had their closed loops for a long time. They had evidently learned to associate the needle punctures with the relief of their distress, so that whenever they began to feel sick they would try in every way they could to call our attention to their desire for another needling, even to the extent of jumping on the table where the procedure was customarily done. Once on the table, such a dog would lie down and could be readily rolled onto its back, lying quietly with paws dangling during the needle puncture. As soon as the withdrawal of fluid had been completed, the dog would jump off the table, frisking and wagging his tail, and then usually would go directly to his food pan and begin to gulp down the meat he had turned from so dispiritedly only a short time previously.

Since 1930, the approximate period I have been writing about, there have been many other demonstrations of the remarkable plasticity of reflex mechanisms, and I wish to interrupt my story at this point to mention two such demonstrations. Arthur Ward and J.G. Dusser de Barenne investigated the changes in a monkey's knee jerks that could be elicited by concurrent electrical stimulation of the motor cortex of the monkey's brain (Dusser de Barenne and Ward 1937). Their report began as follows: "During an investigation on the influence of cortical stimulation on the knee jerk of the narcotized monkey, the rhythmically elicited knee reflexes became gradually weaker for no apparent reason. Suddenly, the animal voided a large quantum of urine, after which the reflexes returned to their previous size. Later on, when the reflexes diminished again, expression of the urinary bladder resulted in a prompt and lasting enhancement of the knee jerks." To investigate this interesting phenomenon, they distended the bladder with water at controlled pressures and recorded the effect on the knee jerk. Individual animals varied somewhat in the promptness with which the inhibition of the skeletal reflex appeared and in the rate of recovery of the usual reflex amplitude after the bladder pressure dropped. Occasionally the amplitude of the knee jerk was temporarily augmented immediately after the pressure was lowered. As to this individual variability, these investigators said, "It seems as if the inhibition is more abrupt in those animals in which the wall of the abdominal organ does not yield readily to the pressure."

A further study of this phenomenon showed that a similar distention of the gall bladder or the small intestine inhibited the knee jerk just as bladder distention did. That the inhibition was not due to some influence descending from the brain was shown by the fact that similar changes in the knee jerk could be elicited by visceral stimulation after experimental animals had recovered from a transection of the spinal cord in the midthoracic region. Since Dusser de Barenne and Ward's article was published, other investigators have reported similar observations. It is now an accepted fact that abnormal degrees of tension acting on hollow viscera can produce widespread changes in skeletal reflexes, usually of an inhibitory type. Whatever the factors that are responsible for such changes, their principal site of action seems to be the gray matter of the spinal cord, that is, within the "internuncial pools" in which reflex circuits are subject to modulation. This information, based on experimental studies, was available before the "gamma efferents" were discovered and before we knew anything about their ability to influence reflex circuits and to modify the motor output resulting from stimulation of the motor cortex. What this all adds up to, of course, is that the old concept of a "simple reflex arc" is gone forever, replaced by a new realization of the dynamic plasticity of neural functioning, not only in the modulation of the motor output but presumably on the sensory input as well.

The other observation that illustrates this dynamic plasticity was made in Tasaki's laboratory at the National Institutes of Health. His collaborator, Dr. Spyropoulos, had consented to demonstrate for me the ability of a single motor neuron to respond to electrical stimulation. For this purpose, he was using a nerve muscle preparation from an adult toad. The motor fibers to the muscle had been divided one by one under a dissecting microscope until only a single fiber remained to connect the muscle bundle and the site for stimulation. Under the microscope I could see the proximal and distal portions of the divided nerve lying in their respective pools of normal saline with only one fiber connecting them, on which two nodes of Ranvier were visible. When a single electrical pulse was delivered to the proximal portion of this fiber a muscle twitch resulted, the electrical effects of which could be recorded on the nearby oscillograph. The point of greatest interest to me was the fact that the single pulse elicited two or more electrical responses. I asked Dr. Spyropoulos why this should be so. He said that ordinarily a single pulse produced only a single response, but the animal he was using was an adult toad and this happened to be the mating season for toads. He reminded me that during this season the male toad often holds the female in a firm clasp for relatively long periods. As long as the mating season lasts, the male toad's neuromuscular mechanisms are altered so that a single pulse always tended to elicit a multiple muscular response. He added that if he put this preparation in salt solution and left it in an incubator overnight, the multiple response would disappear and a single electrical pulse would elicit but one electrical response in the muscle. He interpreted this observation as implying that during the mating season the adult toad must have in its circulation some water-soluble substance that has the power to augment the muscular response to electrical stimulation.

7

Irritative Nerve Lesions

One night about midnight I was awakened by the ringing of my telephone. An agitated young woman was calling to tell me that her husband had just had a massive bowel hemorrhage and was in a state of collapse. Just before getting undressed he had complained of a cramping pain and had hurried to the bathroom. A few minutes later she heard her name called faintly, followed by a thud. She rushed to the bathroom to find him lying unconscious on the floor; his face and hands were white and covered with drops of sweat.

The toilet had not been flushed and the bowl contained much bright red blood. She managed to get him onto a bed but had been afraid to move him enough to take his clothes off. He was now lying across the bed, groaning faintly but not speaking. I told this frightened woman that I would come at once and in the meantime she was not to try to move him but to cover him warmly. I warned her not to flush the toilet because an examination of its contents might give me some estimate of his blood loss. When I arrived at their home I found that the wife had accurately described the man's condition. He lay white and motionless across the bed, conscious but saying nothing. I asked him if he was in much pain and he nodded his head. When I asked him where his pain was worst, he whispered, "all over." He continued to groan faintly while his wife told me more of his story. He had been in excellent health and spirits all evening, and prior to his complaining of the cramping pain he had been sitting quietly, reading and listening to music. She had no suspicion that anything was wrong until he had called her from the bathroom.

When I removed his clothing I found it difficult to make a satisfactory examination because he held himself so rigidly and would not relax when I tried to palpate his abdomen. His groaning increased when I made a rectal examination but I could not tell whether it was because I was hurting him or because he was afraid of what I might find. His pallor, sweating, rapid pulse and low blood pressure combined to suggest a severe loss of blood, but an examination of the contents of the toilet bowl did not support this diagnosis. The water was colored a bright red but was too translucent to suggest fresh blood. When I stirred up the fluid, amidst scanty fecal material there were many fragments that looked like pieces of beets. I asked the wife if he had eaten any beets recently. She said her husband had always been inordinately fond of pickled beets and for lunch had eaten a huge quantity of them and little else. I told her that I believed the red color of the fluid was due to the presence of the beet fragments and that perhaps her husband's condition might be due to fright when he had seen what he thought was blood in the toilet bowl. She smiled in relief and we were both smiling as we walked back into the bedroom. The patient frowned when he saw our expressions and seemed to be offended because we could smile when he was so critically ill. It took some time to convince him that the fluid in the toilet was discolored by beet juice rather than by blood, but after that his condition improved rapidly. Within a half hour he was moving about in his usual energetic fashion and offering to pour me a drink if I would stay and chat.

It may seem strange to open a chapter on "Irritative Nerve Lesions" with this striking example of how closely psychic states can mimic organic disease, pain and all. My reason for doing so is that I wish to register my conviction that there are psychic factors involved in every patient's complaints of pain. Every physician has had patients whose fear of cancer or heart disease has influenced them to describe a pain as severe, only to see the same pain reduced to negligible proportions when their fears have been dispelled. In such cases is easy to say that the pain has not changed but only the patient's reaction to it. But I doubt that this assumption is ever justified and I know that it can lead to serious errors in judgment by the physician who deals with the type of "irritative nerve lesion" I wish to describe. I had occasion to examine many such cases in the 1930s, and here is how it came about.

For eight years, beginning in 1932, I served part time as a medical examiner for the Oregon State Industrial Accident Commission. In company with a few colleagues I spent one day each week at the Commission's offices in Portland, examining injured workers whose cases raised problems for which the commissioners sought medical and surgical advice. There was no need for us to see the great majority of workers whose injuries healed in a normal fashion and who were able to return to work in a reasonable length of time. We saw only those whose progress had not been satisfactory or who disagreed with their attending physicians as to whether they were able to return to work. Among this latter group were a considerable number of men who had sustained partial or complete finger amputations. Over and over I heard this combination of complaints from these men: "The stump is always cold; it is so sensitive I can't bear to let anyone touch it; I can't tolerate any form of physiotherapy; the stump pains me all the time, the ache tending to spread to adjacent fingers or into the whole hand and even the whole arm." This triad of coldness, hypersensitivity, and pain seemed to be characteristic of most finger injuries, whether the loss of tissue was large or small. In fact, I would say that these complaints are present in some degree after all finger injuries, although most soon disappear under physiotherapy treatments and the active use of the hand. But when the pain and hyperesthesia are so excessive that neither use nor physiotherapy can be tolerated, the period of disability tends to be greatly prolonged.

In 1933 I examined a timber feller whose case the commissioners had instructed me to close. More than a year previously this man had cut off the tip of his left thumb with an axe. The wound healed promptly but the scar remained so sensitive that the man was unable to carry on his work after his case had been closed. The commissioners reopened the case when the attending surgeon recommended that the distal phalanx of this man's thumb be removed to provide a better pad over the stump. After this operation the wound healed but the man complained that the stump was more painful and sensitive than ever. In the year that had elapsed since the reamputation, the case had been closed two more times on a "permanent-partial-disability rating," but each time it had had to be reopened again. I was instructed by the commissioners to recommend as generous a disability award as would be consistent with my findings and then to close the case so that it would stay closed.

anything in her left hand, she was liable to drop it unexpectedly. In the meantime, I had received a note from her employer's insurance carrier informing me that this woman had been examined by two other physicians, neither of whom could account for her bizarre complaints. One of them said he thought she was an "out-and-out malingerer."

The scar on her index finger pad was almost invisible, yet the entire finger seemed extremely sensitive, so much so that she wouldn't let me touch it and she jerked her hand away when I blew my breath on it. When she gingerly touched this finger against the thermocouples of a dermamometer, it recorded the temperature of the finger as 4°C lower than that of the right index finger. In fact, the entire left hand appeared slightly cyanotic and edematous and all parts of it measured from one to four degrees colder than the right hand. When I tested the grip of each hand, the contrast in the strength she exhibited on the two sides was so great that I had the impression that she was not even trying to grip with her left hand. She complained of tenderness when I palpated the muscles of her left arm and she protested bitterly when I pressed on her brachial artery. I used a very fine needle to start an injection of procaine solution into the finger but she screamed and struggled to jerk her hand away. However, as soon as the whole finger pad had been expanded with the solution she quieted down and said the whole arm felt better. The finger assumed a brilliant red color and the entire hand became hot. She then demonstrated quite a normal grip with her left hand. I suggested that she had not been trying in the previous test but she denied this and said that when her pain was severe her arm muscles were not only weak but also completely unreliable. When she reported back to my office a week later, she said that the injection had markedly reduced her symptoms and for the first time she could "see hope ahead." Although she dreaded another injection, the first one had had such a good effect that she was willing to submit to any number of injections if I thought they would contribute to her further improvement. She received five injections at weekly intervals, after which she was able to return to work and had no subsequent recurrence of symptoms.

A 38-year-old stenographer was referred to me by her employer with the following story. Eighteen months previously she had been injured in an automobile accident and had been confined to a hospital for six months. In the same accident her fiancé had been killed. They were planning to get married soon and his death, together with the fact that she felt she was getting beyond the marriageable age, had been a source of great grief to her. Since her return to work she had complained of severe headaches, which had caused her to be absent from the office with increasing frequency. Her employer added that she had been a valuable member of his office force but he was afraid he would have to discharge her unless something could be done to relieve her headaches. He told me that he was inclined to agree with the opinion of a previous consultant that her symptoms were all of psychic origin.

This patient told me that she had been confined to a hospital after the accident because she had suffered a bad fracture of her left femur, a fractured jaw, and a laceration over her left eye. The forehead and scalp on the left side remained numb for most of the six months she remained in the hospital but she did not suffer from headaches during this period. When sensation began to return to the numb area, the skin became extremely sensitive and at times gave rise to attacks of intolerable itching. If she yielded to the temptation to scratch the skin, a severe burning sensation supervened and lasted for hours. At times this burning sensation lasted all night and prevented sleep. Coincident with the return of cutaneous sensibility above the scar area, she began to have recurrent, severe headaches. The ache always started in the left frontal region and then spread to both temples, finally involving the whole head. These headaches had increased in frequency and severity. In addition to these complaints she said that she could not lie on her left side without bringing on dizziness and a sensation as if she were revolving in space in a clockwise direction.

The scar over her left eye was partially hidden in the eyebrow hair. Her point of greatest tenderness was over the supraorbital notch, and pressure there started an aching pain over the left forehead and scalp. Tapping lightly over the scar caused prickling paresthesias over this same skin distribution. This area of skin was hyperesthetic, although there was no demonstrable loss of sensory discrimination. When I expanded the scar with procaine solution she complained of severe pain. I made no attempt to inject the nerve beneath the notch, yet the entire distribution of the supraorbital nerve became numb. When she reported to my office a week later, she said she did not care to submit to any more injections because after the local anesthetic effect had worn off, the skin area seemed to be more sensitive than ever. However, she admitted that her headaches and the burning sensation had

8

Glomus Tumors

In 1931 Mrs. M., the wife of a physician, sought my advice about what she called an "injured nerve" in her left little finger. Four years previously she had noticed that this finger was becoming sensitive near the base of the fingernail. She could not recall having injured the finger in any way. At first the sensitivity was apparent only when she happened to strike the finger, but it soon became so tender to pressure that she could not wear a glove or permit the nail to be manicured. Later, she began to have intermittent attacks of "terrible, stabbing pain" lasting for a few seconds and then fading slowly. These attacks increased in severity and frequency. Some days she had only a few; at other times a succession of attacks might occur all day long, "particularly if it was going to rain or change temperature." Recently she had noticed that when the pain was severe, a "bluish, bruised" spot appeared just proximal to the base of the nail on its radial aspect. While the discoloration was present and the pain at its height, she could not tolerate the lightest touch anywhere near the distal phalanx. As the pain subsided, the color changed to red. Often, when the finger pain was intense, she also had pain on the ulnar side of her wrist on its volar aspect and occasionally a tingling pain was felt just above her left clavicle. At times the pain came on at night, waking her from sleep and causing her to walk the floor until it subsided. She was unable to lie on her left side or wear a tight-sleeved dress without precipitating attacks, which were also brought on by exposing the left hand to either heat or cold. Because of the terrible sensitivity of this finger she could do little housework, and she had few social contacts because when she went out

I asked her to stand by with these three syringes, ready for use at any time, while I sat beside the bed watching Nick struggle for breath. I had temporarily forgotten about his phantom symptoms. When it began to appear that he was improving without medication, I remembered to ask him if the injection had modified his pain in any way. He told me that an amazing change had taken place. While I was completing the left-side injection he had felt the phantom hand relax and warm. One by one his fingers had opened and for the first time since his amputation he could move them voluntarily. He said that the whole arm felt "relaxed, warm, and perfectly normal."

While I was completing the left-side injection he had felt the phantom hand relax and warm. One by one his fingers had opened and for the first time since his amputation he could move them voluntarily.

This remarkable change in Nick's symptoms persisted during the two days my wife and I continued our visit in his home. The stump remained warm and relaxed. There was a corresponding change in Nick's mood. He laughed a great deal, kept exclaiming about how good he felt, and he was repeatedly testing his ability to move his phantom fingers. I told Nick that on the basis of this favorable prognostic test I was now willing to perform the sympathetic ganglionectomy. I would make preparations for the operation at my hospital and he was to fly to Portland Sunday morning for surgery on Monday. But Nick failed to show up on the appointed day and when I called him by phone that night to find out why, he could give me no good reason except that he thought he would defer the operation for a while.

Two months later I visited Nick again in his hometown and asked why he was putting off an operation that promised so much relief. He told me that he had been completely free from pain ever since the procaine injection, that the stump was no longer cold and sensitive, and that the phantom hand had remained warm, relaxed, and freely movable. He was grateful for this improvement but more than ever convinced that his pains had been imaginary and that the injection had "proved" he was "just a damned neurasthenic." When I denied this, he demanded to know how the transient effects of procaine could bring about such a persistent change in his symptoms. I told him about some of my cases in which procaine injections had relieved chronic pain states, many of them permanently. I did not know *why* the pain relief had persisted in his case but the fact that it had was enough for me. If his pain recurred another procaine injection might again relieve him for several months, so that we might never have to perform a ganglionectomy.

Nick flew to Portland in September 1934 to tell me he needed another injection. The first one had conferred complete relief of symptoms for some six months, after which the pain began to come back. Finally, all his previous symptoms had returned and a new sensation had been added. He described it as a sensation of terrible constriction in the shoulder "as if a wire tourniquet were being constantly tightened around it." Nick had just returned from a hunting trip in which he had been out shooting pheasants during cold, rainy weather. Although he had worn two woolen socks over the stump, it had become very cold and his pains had become much worse. When I asked Nick why he had not come sooner for a second injection, he had difficulty explaining the psychological factors that had held him back. He said he had never been convinced that his symptoms had any organic basis and he spoke of them as an "obsession" which he thought had been temporarily dispelled by the ordeal of the first injection and some kind of "hocus-pocus" on my part. This line of reasoning had made it difficult for him to believe that a second injection would have a similar beneficial effect. Despite this doubt, he had been able to "kid" himself along by saying, "I can stand the pain today and if it gets worse tomorrow all I will have to do to relieve it is to let Bill inject me again." He knew that this was a frail prop to lean on, yet he dreaded to run the risk of losing it by putting it to a test.

Arrangements were made to give Nick a second procaine injection on a Friday in October, the day before the annual Oregon-Washington football game in Portland, which he and his wife planned to attend. At this session I was careful to inject only the ganglia on the left side.

11

Tentative Interpretations

The cases I have been describing are certainly not common even in the experience of a medical examiner for an industrial accident commission. In the first years of my service in this capacity I saw so few of them and at such long intervals apart that they made little impression on me except that they were "not according to Hoyle." The complaints of these patients seemed to be excessive in relation to any cause I could identify. Their symptoms did not remain confined to the distribution of any single somatic nerve or spinal segment, and in some cases they spread beyond the injured limb to other extremities or distant internal organs. The men often complained of tenderness over blood vessels or over muscles at a distance from the site of injury and some said the muscles of the affected limb were no longer dependable in their functioning. If I tested the grip strength of an affected hand, the dynamometer reading was so much lower than for the normal hand that I had the impression the man was deliberately trying to exaggerate his disability. In some cases the man's attitude was prejudicial in that he seemed either bellicose or overly defensive. He might also show signs of nervousness such as excessive sweating, tremor, and rapid pulse. When the factor of compensation and perhaps pressure from the commissioners to close the case were added to all of this, it was easy to conclude that the complaints had no organic basis and to label the case with some such title as "psychasthenia," "hysteria," "compensation neurosis," or "malingering."

Peculiarly enough, however, when a medical examiner encounters these same unusual features in a full-blown case of "Volkmann's is-

chemic paralysis," "Sudeck's atrophy," or "causalgia," the organic basis for the patient's complaints is not questioned. These are well-recognized clinical syndromes that have been described by famous clinicians and the descriptions appear in every modern textbook dealing with trauma. Furthermore, in these classical syndromes the physical evidence of vasomotor, sudomotor, and trophic changes in the affected limb are so profound that they cannot be overlooked. These physical signs point toward some serious derangement of function in the centers within the nervous system that regulate the physiology of the limb. The ultimate source of this dysfunction is not known but its organic nature is obvious and no one seems to doubt that these classical pain syndromes are real.

It may seem strange that the organic nature of these major syndromes should be so universally recognized while lesser degrees of what seems to be an essentially similar process are so often assumed to be of purely psychic origin, yet this is so. I know that it took a long time and many cases to convince me that the bizarre pattern of signs and symptoms I was observing in some of the injured workers must have an organic basis and was mechanistically related to other "causalgic states." My association with my fellow medical examiners and other colleagues older and wiser than I helped me to reach this interpretation. Once I did, I understood my job better and became a more reliable witness in representing the interests of both the insured workers and the commissioners. To understand this it might help if I gave a brief description of the major assignments the Oregon State Industrial Accident Commissioners passed on to their medical examiners.

In general, the function of the examiners was to give the commissioners advice in two types of cases. In the first group were the cases that were ready for closure, and the principal question at issue was whether the injured worker had any residual disability that could be assumed to be permanent and would entitle him to receive a monetary reward according to the state law under which the commission operated. In many instances the worker had lost a finger, a hand, a foot, or perhaps a whole arm as a result of an accident. As specified by the law, the highest award for a "permanent partial disability" that could be paid, or any loss, was based on the "total loss of an arm" and was a fixed sum of money. The law also specified that the loss of each part of the body represented a definite percentage of this total. We examiners were provided with a schedule showing the percentage for each type of loss. The only reason the commissioners wanted the advice of their medical examiners before granting the prescribed award in each case was that in particular instances there might be factors present that warranted a somewhat larger award than the law provided. When the evaluation of such factors was difficult we examiners could consult with one another, but in general, the task of closing cases was not difficult and we usually carried it out in a more or less automatic fashion.

The second major assignment for the examiners was to advise the commissioners as to further treatment needed by workers whose cases were not ready for closure. This was always a difficult task and though we might consult with each other as to the proper recommendation in particular cases, there were many types of pain syndrome that we admittedly did not understand. Included in this category were such commonplace conditions as "post-traumatic headache," "bad backs," "painful scars," "whiplash injuries of the neck," "painful feet," and the full range of major and minor "causalgias." We spoke of such conditions as our *bêtes noires* and frequently asked each other such questions as these: How can a simple 'catch' in a man's back muscles, incurred in the performance of his regular work and which has been experienced many times previously without ever causing serious aftereffects, now give rise to so much pain and disability that he is not able to resume work for months or years? . . . What makes one surgical scar so exquisitely sensitive while hundreds of similar scars heal promptly and without residual symptoms? . . . How can a sudden jerk of a man's head, which produces no visible bone or joint injury, cause him such severe neck pain and so many other widespread complaints? . . . In what way does an injury to sensory nerve fibers followed by the development of a major causalgia differ from apparently similar nerve injuries that cause little or no pain? I don't mean to imply that we ever debated these particular questions in any formal manner; there seemed to be little point in spending a lot of time on problems for which none of us had answers. Nevertheless, questions of this kind were in the backs of our minds as we discussed problem cases, and the closest we ever came to answering them was to say that in certain instances the injury to sensory nerve fibers gave rise to a persistent source of irritation while in other instances it did not. As to what the nature of this "irritation" might be, we had no way of knowing.

In 1938 I wrote two articles under the title "Post-traumatic Pain Syndromes" in which I reported ten cases and discussed the various problems they raised (Livingston 1938a,b). I have included the full "Discussion" in Appendix A. As I read it now, it seems a bit labored and wordy so in this chapter I am reproducing only the final section, "A Suggested Interpretation," because it indicates the direction of my thinking at that time.

A Suggested Interpretation

I am reluctant to commit to writing my present interpretation of the pathological physiology which these cases represent. The reluctance is increased by the realization that it does not conform to some of the accepted interpretations of pain phenomena, and by my lack of experimental evidence obtained under the rigid control conditions prevailing in the research laboratory. But I have already said enough to indicate my trend of thought regarding these cases and to make it necessary to attempt a more complete formulation of these concepts. In discussing the same type of case in a former writing (Livingston 1935, p. 214) I said, "It seems probable that the injury to certain tissues starts a cumulative process which is not confined to a single nerve distribution and which tends to spread to involve the spinal cord in diffuse reflex phenomena in which the sympathetic nerves are prominently affected. Today I would reaffirm that statement, but would broaden its application."

After any injury, reflexes immediately begin to exert their influences upon the affected area. Some of the reflexes are a fundamental component of the organism's defense mechanisms and contribute to the repair process. Others may actually prolong disability. In the great majority of cases of injury, the color changes, hyperesthesia, sensitiveness to cold, and other phenomena so frequently observed, tend to disappear spontaneously with the completion of the healing process. But in other instances an irritative process persists. As with causalgia, there are probably nerve fibers involved in scar or subjected to some form of constant stimulation. In the cases under discussion in this paper, the nerve fibers may not be part of a major nerve, but instead may be minute units in the walls of blood vessels, in the skin or in the deeper tissues. Again, as with causalgia, these irritated nerve fibers are capable of initiating a vicious circle of reflexes. The original lesion acts as a trigger point to set off a series of reflex changes which gradually dominate the clinical picture and obscure the origin. As the train of symptoms gathers momentum and cord segments become secondarily involved, it may become increasingly difficult to stop. The hyperesthesia which develops adds new pain impulses, the vasomotor phenomena may interfere with nutrition over a wider area and lead to new tissue changes, in themselves capable of initiating other reflexes. And so the vicious circle grows in scope and force until it has created a clinical picture out of all proportion to the original lesion. Even the removal of the trigger point may not entirely abolish the secondary harmful effects of the process. But in other instances, once the trigger point ceases to contribute its irritative influence, the process may subside and its force be dissipated.

Since the whole process seems to be ultimately dependent upon nerve reflexes, one may undertake treatment by interrupting these nerve impulses with procaine solution. A single injection may lessen the momentum of the vicious circle but may not stop it. Repeated injections may gradually narrow its scope and check its force. When the trigger point cannot be located one may sometimes alleviate the condition by interrupting the sympathetic component of the syndrome, and with part of the circle interrupted, normal healing processes may complete the cure.

This concept is highly theoretical and may not stand critical analysis, but at least it affords a rationale for a method of treatment which may be worthy of further trial.

(*Western Journal of Surgery, Obstetrics and Gynecology* 1938b; 46:433–434).

12

Missile Wounds of Nerves

T he manuscript for *Pain Mechanisms* was completed late in 1941 and was sent to the medical editor of the Macmillan Company. He acknowledged its receipt after which there was a long period of silence. Then a letter came saying that he had sent the manuscript to a neurosurgeon for an expert opinion as to its merit, and after a careful reading, this consultant had advised him not to publish it. The letter contained excerpts from the consultant's report to the effect that the interpretations I had expressed in the manuscript were "purely speculative," "unorthodox," and its publication would "probably do more harm than good." I was asked for comments. My first comments were unprintable and I did not send them on. I finally wrote that I could understand why a neurosurgeon might not like the interpretations, as they were frankly speculative and controversial, but I felt that they gave a more dynamic concept of pain than did orthodox interpretations, which I was convinced were too rigid and mechanistic. One of my purposes in writing the book was to advance a tentative interpretation that would invite discussion and perhaps would eventually be put to experimental testing. The editor thanked me for my comments and again there followed months of silence.

In the meantime, the possibility of war with Japan was looming and I had enlisted in the Naval Medical Corps Reserve. The captain of the Thirteenth Naval District had told me that in the event of war my services would be needed to care for the peripheral nerve injuries and pain problems of wounded men. He asked me to organize "Neurosurgical Unit No. 104," which would consist of myself, two neurosurgeons, a nurse-anesthetist, and an instrument nurse.

The plan was to fly this team and its special equipment from one naval hospital to another on the mainland to care for the nerve-injury cases being brought in from combat areas in the South Pacific. This assignment delighted me because I knew that if war came I wanted to be in it and this unit would afford a unique opportunity to study one type of war wound intensively. I was aware, too, that most of what was known about the care of peripheral nerve wounding had been learned during a war period by such men as Mitchell, Tinel (1918), Leriche, and Pollock and Davis (1933). So, I happily went about completing the organization of this proposed specialty unit. Two well-qualified neurosurgeons were signed up and I managed to persuade two exceptionally efficient nurses to join the group on the understanding that we would be called into service as a surgical team.

My wife and I were out driving in our car and listening to radio music on that Sunday afternoon in December 1941, when the voice of President Roosevelt broke in to tell the story of the tragic attack on Pearl Harbor. I said to my wife, "Well, this is it," and my immediate impulse was to kiss her goodbye, step out of the car, and gallop off to war. Instead, I waited for weeks and months for my orders to active duty. In the meantime, one by one the other members of Neuro-surgical Unit No. 104 were called into service and I never saw but one of them during the entire war period. Finally, on my birthday in October 1942 I received two telegrams. One was from the Macmillan editor saying that my manuscript was being accepted for publication. The other was from the Surgeon General's Office, ordering me to active duty in the Oakland Naval Hospital in California. Both messages pleased me, although I assumed that the book would probably never be published because I expected that by the time I should have been correcting galley and page proofs and preparing an index I would probably be out on some south sea island. However, as things worked out I remained on duty at the Oakland Naval Hospital for the duration of the war, so I had no real difficulty in completing the final details relating to the book.

My first year of service in the navy was both disappointing and frustrating as well as a period of hard work. At that time our hospital consisted of a scattered group of frame buildings on Oak Knoll in the outskirts of Oakland. The capacity was some 400 beds and the hospital served as a clearing station for the disabled marines and sailors brought to the port of San Francisco by ship convoys. Our cases had to be shipped out almost as fast as they came in, so there was little time to study individual cases and still complete the oceans of paper work. It seemed that I would have little to do with peripheral nerve injuries as there was already a ward for neurosurgical cases with two competent neurosurgeons in charge. I was assigned to general surgery and put in charge of a forty-bed ward that seemed to be filled with patients with fractured bones, flat feet, or bad backs. At first my contact with peripheral nerve cases was limited to the few I could beg, borrow, or steal from other wards. But as it became known that I was willing to attack any kind of pain problem, I began to collect more and more cases of major and minor causalgia on my ward and the neurosurgeons didn't seem to object to my keeping them. And it so happened that during the time I was correcting galley proofs of the chapter in which I had copied Weir Mitchell's dramatic report of one of his cases of causalgia, I had on my own ward three cases that were every bit as striking as Mitchell's had been.

Conditions changed rapidly during the second year as the convoys brought in drafts of wounded men numbering in the hundreds and sometimes in the thousands. The hospital capacity was greatly expanded and finally reached some 12,000 beds. It was soon evident that there were too many cases of peripheral nerve injury for any single ward to accommodate, so the neurosurgeons took over the cases with head injuries, while I looked after the nerve cases. Eventually, our hospital was designated as one of four naval centers for the study and treatment of peripheral nerve injuries. I acquired a staff of medical officers that included general surgeons, neurosurgeons, neurologists, and psychiatrists and a number of young men sent to us for training in nerve surgery. Before the war was over our cases filled four or five wards and our staff settled down to a hard-working and enthusiastic team. We maintained detailed case histories on all of our patients in addition to the regular hospital records, so that we gradually accumulated a valuable fund of information relating to all types of peripheral nerve injury. We made punch cards for our cases so that we could quickly estimate percentages of each type of problem they presented. I still have in my possession 1279 of these detailed case histories recorded during my period of service; 919 of these were cases of nerve injury due to wounding by high-velocity missiles, so we were able to make statistical analyses of the various phenomena associated with this type of wounding.

As peripheral nerves are such sensitive structures and the carriers of all sensory impressions, it would be natural to expect that missile wounds of nerves would be the most painful of all wounds. Instead, our records indicated that severe pain is the exception rather than the rule in such cases. Approximately 70% of our patients stated flatly that they had experienced no pain of any consequence at the time of wounding and none directly referable to the injured nerve during their period of convalescence. Less than 20% of the men claimed to have experienced severe pain from the moment of wounding. Sometimes this pain was limited to the site of wounding; more often it was referred distally into the hand or foot and occasionally it seemed to involve the entire limb. Most of the men reported that they had felt the impact of the missile, although a few had not known they were hit until they saw their own blood running or they lost control of the injured limb. Almost never did a patient report that he had any sense of penetration as the missile traversed parts of his body. The sensation of impact was usually compared to being hit a heavy blow with some blunt object, such as a baseball bat, hard enough to numb the entire extremity. Occasionally, the sensation of impact was compared to an electric shock or a bee sting.

There were two principal reasons why we recorded a detailed report of each man's experiences at the time he was hit by a high-velocity missile. One was that we thought that perhaps the psychic trauma due to wounding might have something to do with the severity of the man's subsequent symptoms and the duration of his disability. The other reason was that we hoped to get clues as to how the central nervous system responded to massive stimulation. As to the first objective, if the wounding per se had anything to do with the subsequent progress of the case, our records failed to show it. However, the records did bring out a number of interesting facts. In some instances, the men actually welcomed their wounds as representing a means of escape from conditions they felt were increasingly intolerable, as on Guadalcanal. To them a wound meant rest, protection, and perhaps a return home. Many of the men said they would gladly have "settled" for a serious wound if only they could have been sure that it would not kill them or cause too much suffering. Their fears seemed to take two forms—fear of death and suffering and fear of showing their fear to others. Some were sustained by an "it can't happen to me" feeling that young people generally share, although the older marines with considerable battle experience had adopted a fatalistic attitude in saying they expected to "get it when their number was up."

They had also learned that bullet wounds are usually surprisingly free from pain and they would often tell some wounded man who cried when he was hit to "pipe down." But the less experienced young men somehow did not expect to die or to be wounded, so that the most common sensation they experienced at the time of wounding was surprise. They did not always use the same word in describing this reaction, yet the words "astonished," "surprised," "amazed," and "dumbfounded" occurred with great frequency in our records. Associated with such words were descriptions of behavior suited to them. For example, a young marine is crawling through the grass toward a Japanese position when a grenade explodes nearby. He is momentarily stunned and when he opens his eyes he sees a man's hand lying on the ground a few inches from his face. He thinks, "Some poor devil has lost an arm," and then he sees a ring on the hand, which he recognizes as his own. At the same moment he becomes aware that his left arm has "gone." "My God, that's mine," he thinks and sits up. As he moves, the hand drags toward him but he is afraid to stand up for fear the arm will fall from his sleeve. There he sits, in the line of fire, pulling on the arm to make sure it is still attached to his body or manipulating its fingers with his normal hand while wondering why he is unable to arouse any feeling or movement in them.

Before I describe three types of "physiological" responses to wounding, I might mention some of the experimental work that was available to us at that time. The destructive potential of a speeding bullet is dependent upon many factors such as its velocity, mass, shape, hardness, its "tumble" or oscillation in flight, its angle of incidence, and the density of the tissues it traverses. The experts have a complex formula for calculating this potential but a good working rule is that the destructive potential varies as the first power of the mass and the cube of the velocity. Thus, increasing the mass of a bullet three times would triple its destructive force, while increasing its velocity three times would make its destructive power nine times greater. Incidentally, the rifles that the Japanese soldiers used on Guadalcanal were lighter than our own but the muzzle velocity of their bullets was considerably higher. As a bullet passes through living tissue it releases its enormous store of kinetic energy in proportion to its rate of slowing. Everyone knows how rapidly water slows the speed of a bullet, and as human tissues are composed largely of water, the rate of slowing is comparable. Experimental studies on animals have made it possible to visualize some of the tissue effects due to the passage of a bullet. By using movie cameras and a surge-type of X-ray it is possible to record exposures as short as a millisecond or to take hundreds of successive frames per second of a dog's leg through which a bullet has been fired from a high-power rifle. Serial pictures of the leg show that after the bullet has passed completely through the limb, it swells to an enormous size two or three times in succession. X-ray pictures indicate that the swelling phases are due to successive cavitations within the tissues and it is during these sudden expansions that bones may fracture and tissues are disrupted, even when these structures may be some distance away from the actual path of the missile. The tissue destruction is comparable to that which would be produced by exploding a charge of TNT deep inside the limb. Under these circumstances, it is not surprising that nerves should be massively stimulated or paralyzed whether or not the missile strikes them directly.

Our records indicated that when peripheral nerves are injured by high-velocity missiles the muscles of the injured limbs customarily exhibit a flaccid paralysis, yet a careful history of the events immediately following the wounding indicates that the paralysis is often preceded by nerve stimulation. We studied three phenomena that were attributed to nerve stimulation: involuntary movements, hallucinations of posture, and transient paraplegia. Each deserves a brief comment and can be illustrated by a single case history.

About 30% of our patients wounded by high-velocity missiles reported that they had observed some involuntary movement of the limb at the time of wounding. After eliminating all the cases in which the limb movement might have been mechanical and those in which the muscular movement was limited to a contraction into the palm of the ring and little fingers, there remained slightly more than 16% of the cases in which the movement suggested a definite period of nerve stimulation. In most of these cases the muscular movement was clonic or took the form of a sustained muscular contraction, but in rare instances such as the one I will describe, the movement involved limbs on the opposite side of the body from the site of wounding.

A marine private was wounded by mortar shell fragments during the fighting on Iwo Jima. He was getting up on one knee when the shell exploded about ten yards behind him and to his left. He sustained wounds of the upper left arm and the left thigh. The force of the explosion flung his left arm behind his head, from which position it was retrieved by the medical corpsman who rendered first aid a few minutes later. For a period of five to ten minutes there were forceful, clonic movements of the arm and leg on the right, *unwounded* side, which he thought were similar to those occurring during an epileptic fit. When these movements subsided he seemed to have normal control over both his right extremities, whereas there was neither sensory nor motor function in the left arm and leg for five days. Then motor control gradually came back and at the end of five months his only neurological residuals were a paralysis of the left musculocutaneous nerve in his left arm and of the peroneal nerve in his left leg.

The number of men who reported transient hallucinations of posture was low but these cases were of interest because their sensations were reminiscent of the "phantom limb" phenomena reported by amputees. In these reports the wounded man did not have the impression that the wounded limb was "gone," but it seemed to be in some position quite different from its actual position. Occasionally, this hallucination was associated with the sense of movement in the misplaced limb or the feeling that it was alternately swelling and contracting. A marine sergeant was shot by a bullet that passed through his right brachial plexus during the fighting on Tinian. All sensory and motor function in this arm was abolished for several months. Immediately after the bullet struck him and for about three-quarters of an hour thereafter, he had the feeling that the limb had been "shot off" at the shoulder. Then he began to have phantom sensations in the hand and arm. It felt to him that the arm was extended at his side and the hand was alternately opening and closing with great force "as if it was trying to grab something." He looked down along the side of his body as he lay on a stretcher, but failed to see the hand. He asked the marine who was lying on the next stretcher, "What in hell is my hand grabbing for?" He was told that his right hand was lying quietly across his chest. He kept asking, "Aren't my fingers moving?" Despite assurances to the contrary and his own visual and tactile confirmation of the actual state of the hand, he continued to experience for an hour or more the feeling that the hand was alternately opening and closing despite his efforts to stop the movement.

Some of our patients reported that immediately after wounding they experienced a transient quadriplegia. We did not include in this group the cases that had evidence of a direct injury to the central nervous system in which the quadriplegia persisted for long periods nor those who had lasting neurological residuals. We used the word "transient" as meaning an interval of time measured in seconds or minutes. Four percent of our cases reported that after being hit they had been paralyzed from the neck down for a brief interval, after which function promptly returned in all but the most seriously injured member. This phenomenon occurred most frequently when the wound involved the brachial plexus. In an analysis of 100 cases in which a bullet had seriously damaged the brachial plexus, there were fourteen cases of transient paraplegia. These men were not rendered unconscious and they remained aware of where they were and what was going on around them. They could see and hear and understand what was said to them. Most thought they could move their eyes and could talk but their bodies seemed to have completely disappeared, leaving "only a head."

A 19-year-old marine was hit by a sniper's bullet while walking bent forward through the jungle on Guadalcanal. The bullet entered the posterior triangle of his neck on the right side and emerged over his left scapula. He was "suddenly jerked erect." The movement was involuntary and he reported, "I couldn't prevent it though I knew the sniper might hit me again." He remained stiffly erect for a few seconds and then "the strength seemed to drain out of me and I fell forward on my face." He remained conscious and was aware of no pain except in his face where it had been scratched by the shrubbery during his fall. He reported that he could not move a muscle and for a few seconds was unable to make a sound. Then he suddenly regained his voice and "began to holler." His buddy crawled over to him and asked him where he had been hit. He answered, "I don't know but for Christ's sake roll me off my face." Soon after he had been rolled over, he regained the ability to move his legs and left arm and managed to crawl for a short distance. By the time stretcher bearers reached him he had regained normal control of his limbs except for the right arm, which remained paralyzed for several weeks.

The characteristic features of these cases were: (1) a sudden, complete loss of sensory and motor function in all four extremities, (2) a retention of consciousness and orientation, and (3) a sudden return of function after a brief interval in all parts except the most seriously injured limb. We classified these as cases of "spinal concussion" and thought that the mechanisms producing them might be similar to the mechanisms causing "cerebral concussion." We searched the literature dealing with experimental studies of cerebral concussion and examined the hypothetical explanations offered to account for it to see how they might apply to our cases of spinal concussion. The hypothesis we most favored was one that had been advanced by Walker, Kollros, and Case (1944), who said, "Trauma adequate for concussion causes first an initial excitation with massive discharge of the neurons of the central nervous system, followed by an after-discharge. This results in extinction of the central nervous activity with a decrease in the observable reflex phenomena."

13

A Case of Major Causalgia

O
ne day in June 1945, a member of my staff said to me, "You really ought to go down to Ward 53 to see the young chap just admitted with a diagnosis of 'hysteria.' He is the saddest-looking specimen I have ever seen. In fact, he looks like a spanked spaniel and he cries when you even point toward his foot. He is continually apologizing for his behavior and saying 'my pain is probably all in my head'. I wish you would go see this boy and tell me your impressions." I found "Lee" sitting on the side of his bed with his right foot in a pail of water and a moist rag in his hands. He was badly in need of a haircut, his blonde hair being extremely long and unkempt. When I asked him why he didn't have his hair cut and freshen up a bit, he burst into tears and said he "couldn't stand it." He said he didn't want to talk about his pain or have any more doctors examine him. To divert him I asked him to tell me exactly how he happened to be wounded. He told me the following story readily enough.

Lee's first and only combat experience had been on Okinawa. On April 26 his platoon was moving up toward the Japanese lines. It was raining and the men were strung out in single file along a ridge. A machine gun suddenly opened up on them from a Japanese ambush on their right flank. Lee heard the chatter of the gun and saw men ahead of him fall as the fire swept back along the line.

He ran for a shell hole but was hit in the right leg just before he reached it. He felt the impact as a heavy blow that paralyzed his leg. He dived into the hole, with the leg dragging uselessly behind him. He felt no pain at this time. He was aware that the right foot felt "warm"

103

while the rest of his body felt wet and miserably cold. Stretcher bearers reached him within fifteen minutes and a corpsman gave him an injection of morphine and dressed his wound. The bullet had entered just above and behind the head of the fibula and emerged on the inner aspect of the thigh about four inches higher. Lee was taken by stretcher to the company aid station and then to an army hospital. After a few days he was moved to the hospital ship *Solace*.

His pain did not begin until the second day. It started as a tingling, burning sensation in the foot. At no time did he complain of pain at the site of the wound. By the time he reached the hospital ship the burning pain in the foot had become "unbearable." It was greatly aggravated when he took a deep breath, touched dry objects with his hands, or slid his normal foot down between the sheets; any vibration or sudden noise drove him "crazy." The attendants on the ship could not believe that these complaints were real and they finally refused to give him any more morphine, but they found the only way they could stop his crying was to permit him to keep his foot in a pail of water. Lee was put ashore in Naval Hospital 19 on Tinian for a week or two. While he was there a medical officer had injected something into the nerve above the knee, which relieved his pain completely for about twenty-four hours, but this procedure was not repeated. He was next transferred to a hospital at Pearl Harbor where the doctors injected something into his back. The needles hurt him a great deal and he related that the procedure "scared the wits out of me." However, he admitted that the pain had never again recurred in its original intensity after this injection. Early in June he was flown to the mainland and he noted that his pain was greatly relieved while the plane was flying at a high altitude but it had recurred when the plane began to descend. Lee told me that he thought he was gradually getting better and he felt reasonably comfortable if he could keep the foot in cool water and did not have to touch dry objects with his hands. He was willing to let us explore the wound area but he didn't want an operation on his back or to be given any more injections there.

By the time he had finished his story, Lee had quieted down enough so that I thought he might let me examine his foot. However, he would lift his foot out of the water only if I promised not to touch it. The foot was reddened and the skin was macerated due to long immersion. A small area near the medial malleolus had been denuded and he thought

*He said his pain was made worse
when he saw patients scuffling,
heard a plane flying overhead,
watched anyone walk across the
polished floor on crutches,
or when a door slammed.*

perhaps he had scraped the skin off while asleep. The hyperesthesia was extreme. It involved all of the foot except for a patch near the heel that was hypesthetic. The knee joint was stiffened and any effort to extend the leg was strongly resisted by the muscles. The bullet wounds were well healed and Lee had no complaints referred to them. His pain was described as a terrible burning sensation, mostly confined to the sole of the foot, together with an aching, tingling sensation along the inner border of the sole.

I told Lee that I believed everything he had told me and was confident that his pain wasn't all in his head. We would do everything we could to make him better and our first move would be to start whirlpool baths for the leg. No one would be permitted to touch the temperature and agitation controls but him and he would find that as the water friction gradually increased it would make his foot feel better. If he wanted to get well fast he should cooperate in doing exercises to straighten out his knee, take more exercise out of bed, and begin weight bearing just as soon as possible. He said he would try. However, when it came time to do any of these things, Lee would sob and say he simply had to get his foot back in the water. When the ward officer insisted that he get up on crutches to take some exercise each day, it was necessary to have someone with him every minute to prevent him from going right back to bed. He would hobble through the ward and down the ramp on his crutches, with the leg held high above the floor, crying at the top of his voice, and his wails would continue until he was safely back in the bed with his foot in the pail of water. When movies were shown on the ward, Lee would cover up his head.

When music was loud anywhere near him, he put his fingers in his ears. He said his pain was made worse when he saw patients scuffling, heard a plane flying overhead, watched anyone walk across the polished floor on crutches, or when a door slammed. He would not touch the pages of a book or a newspaper unless his fingers had first been moistened and he flatly refused to have his hair cut. However, when it was quiet and dark on the ward at night, Lee would often get out of bed, carefully moisten the inside of a pair of tennis shoes, slide his wet feet into them, and prowl around the ward for an hour or more. I never saw him do this but I was told by the night nurse that except for a slight limp, he got around on the bad foot surprisingly well. I asked Lee why he couldn't do the same thing in the daytime and he said, "there is too much going on then." I encouraged him to do as much light exercise as possible.

An exploration of the wound area showed the tibial division of the sciatic nerve to be enlarged and firmly fixed in a highly vascular mass of scar tissue. The peroneal portion of the nerve seemed to be relatively intact. Electrical stimulation of the nerve above the knee level elicited good muscle responses in the lower leg and foot. Because the sciatic is such an important nerve and had evidently retained so much of its function, we hesitated to resect the neuroma at this operation. During distention of the nerve with normal saline, it seemed that the posterior half of the trunk was much more resistant to the fluid than the anterior half. The trunk was temporarily covered with a tantalum sleeve because it was impossible to transplant it outside the scar area. This operation completely relieved Lee's pain for a few days. When it did recur, he said it seemed less intense than before the operation, and he certainly seemed to tolerate his physiotherapy treatments better. Lee was sufficiently encouraged by his improvement to permit us to do a procaine block of his right lumbar sympathetic ganglia. The two needles slipped into place easily and just enough procaine solution was injected to produce a warming of the foot, after which 2 cc of 95% alcohol was injected through each needle.

The following day I met Lee walking down the ramp without his crutches. He was wearing a pair of marine shoes for the first time and he carried a large bag of laundry over his shoulder. He said he was on the way to Ships Service to make some purchases and have his hair cut. He told me that the injection in his back had produced a "miracle." It began right while he was on the operating table, with the warming of the foot, when the pain and sensitivity simply "vanished." The improvement persisted and in the following weeks we saw an astonishing change in his disposition. He had never been popular among the men on his ward and they evidently regarded him as being a chronic complainer and mentally dull. Now he was accepted by them and he went with them eagerly to attend movies or out on liberty. Lee returned from a two-month leave of absence to say that he had not had the slightest recurrence of his pain. His only residual symptom was a tingling sensation in the foot if he stamped it hard against the floor. The tantalum sleeve was removed from the nerve trunk and a further course of physiotherapy was given to strengthen his muscles and fully extend the leg. He was returned to duty eleven months from the time of wounding, at which time the only residual was a slight hypesthesia under the right heel and along the medial aspect of his sole.

It is easy to understand why anyone who had never before seen a case of major causalgia might think that Lee was hysterical. Why did he cry so much when he didn't have his foot in a pail of water? Why did he refuse to let the barber cut his hair or make any attempt himself to comb it properly? Why did he shut himself off from the normal activities of the ward by covering his eyes when movies were shown, by putting his fingers in his ears to shut out noise, and by refusing to touch anything dry unless he first moistened his fingers? How can a nerve injury in a single extremity give rise to such a generalized hypersensitivity? No one has ever been able to answer questions of this kind beyond saying that these are the characteristic features of every full-blown case of causalgia. Nor does anyone know what part the sympathetic nervous system may play in sustaining the syndrome, beyond saying that a sympathectomy often cures it. One surgeon who wrote quite a bit about causalgia during this era asserted this dictum: "If a sympathectomy doesn't cure it, it is not a case of causalgia."

In our study of nerve injuries at the Oakland Naval Hospital we encountered relatively few cases of major causalgia. In the total series of 1279 cases only 185 showed any of the signs and symptoms we ascribed to "irritative nerve lesions," and of this group only 33 cases were classified as major causalgia. We performed a sympathectomy on only 11 of these and in two instances the operation failed to confer a satisfactory degree of pain relief. The remaining 22 cases of causalgia did not seem to need a surgical sympathectomy because they made satisfactory improvement under other forms of treatment. I shall speak of this regimen of treatment and the philosophy behind it in a moment, but first I want to say something about the so-called "artificial synapse," which in those days was widely held to be the cause of this syndrome.

In laboratory experiments, Granit and his co-workers had demonstrated that when a sensory nerve is injured or tightly compressed, the individual nerve fibers tend to lose their normal insulation so that nerve impulses can pass directly from one fiber to another at the site of this "artificial synapse" (Granit and Skoglund 1945). Further experiments showed that this "cross-talk" or "short-circuiting" of the nerve impulses was more likely to affect sensory fibers than motor fibers and to involve the smallest fibers more than the larger ones. Based on these findings certain clinicians attempted to account for the syndrome of causalgia. Their arguments went like this: Because the tonic outflow of impulses from the sympathetic nervous system involves very small vasomotor fibers, the artificial synapse permits impulses from these fibers to pass directly into the smallest of the sensory fibers, that is, the "C" fibers that are supposed to be specifically adapted for carrying "burning pain." Thus, the artificial synapse could give rise to the burning pain that characterized causalgia. This interpretation is supported by the fact that a sympathectomy usually cures the syndrome.

The nice thing about this hypothesis is that it seems to be based on experimental evidence. However, the experimental observations do not fit with clinical observations. According to the laboratory findings every nerve injury of any consequence should create an artificial synapse and the cross-firing occurs immediately. Then, as the fibers seal themselves off, the cross-firing diminishes and any sensory disturbances it may have caused would be expected to fade spontaneously. However, few nerve injuries are followed by the development of a causalgia; the onset of pain may be immediate or it may be delayed for hours, days, or even weeks; the resection of the damaged segment of nerve sometimes establishes a cure, whereas it would certainly create a new artificial synapse; the symptoms of causalgia do not remain confined to the distribution of the injured nerve; and finally, even a sympathectomy may fail to cure the causalgic syndrome.

Whatever part the artificial synapse may play in producing the symptomatology associated with normal wound healing, it is obviously not the sole source of the causalgic state. Some additional factor must be present in these cases, which is the power to create and maintain a state of pathological activity within the central nervous system. We called this unknown factor "irritation" and we assumed that it must act on sensory nerve fibers to initiate a sustained barrage of afferent impulses that poured into internuncial pools within the spinal cord and to so disturb their function that both their sensory input and motor output were persistently distorted. The organic nature of the source for the "irritation" was suggested by the fact that in rare instances the removal of some foreign body such as a fragment of steel might be followed by a subsidence of the causalgic state. Otherwise, we were left entirely in the dark as to what the source of the irritation might be so that our treatment of a case of causalgia consisted of efforts to quiet down the central perturbation by any means we could think up. In addition to procaine injections of suspected trigger areas and various types of nerve block, we initiated a regimen of physiotherapy aimed at establishing a normal use of the affected limb. The usual forms of physiotherapy, such as heat, massage, and exercise were ruled out by patients as being intolerable. However, most of our patients obtained a considerable degree of pain relief when the limb was immersed in water, so it was not difficult to persuade them to spend an hour or more each day with the affected part suspended in a whirlpool bath. We always started such treatments without any agitation of the water and we let the patient adjust the water temperature to his liking. No one else was permitted to touch the controls, but the patient was instructed to increase the water agitation as fast as his pain would permit. When he could tolerate the full force of the water agitation he was asked to begin gentle massage and manipulation of the digits under water. When he could tolerate vigorous underwater stimulation, he was to try to carry out the same manipulations out of the water bath. When such a patient reached the stage at which he could permit someone else to administer the treatments, we could assure him that he was well on the road to full recovery and that if he would now begin to use the limb to the extent of his ability, he would almost certainly never have to submit to a surgical sympathectomy.

The philosophy behind this regimen of treatment used at Oak Knoll is the same that underlies all forms of physiotherapy designed to restore function to a disabled limb. We tried to express it by saying, "If you expect to establish a normal output (i.e., restore the normal local physiology) you must first provide a normal input." Of course, a causalgic hand is so exquisitely sensitive that the patient constantly tries to protect it from all forms of stimulation, often wrapping it in wet cloths to avoid even air current stimulation. But we felt that this guarding was "fostering the central bad habits" and our problem was to find forms of stimulation that were gentle enough to be tolerated and then work up from there toward full use of the hand. In our experience, this regimen seemed to produce as good results as did a surgical sympathectomy. We had no strong prejudice against this operation and we did not hesitate to use it if the patient did not respond favorably to what we considered to be a more physiological method of treatment.

To compare any central disturbance of regulatory function to a bad habit may sound farfetched but I think there is some justification for using this simile. "Dis-use" seems to throw the central regulatory mechanisms out of kilter very readily and this seems to hold true whether one is talking about muscles that have been long immobilized on splints, people trying to walk normally after a long stay in bed, astronauts recovering from periods of weightlessness, athletes trying to "get back in condition" after a brief break in training, or such mundane subjects as bowel regularity. On the other side of this coin, as I see it, is the amazing capacity of many body tissues to increase their resistance to reiterated trauma. Hands seem to "toughen up" after a few days of using a shovel or playing hand-ball; a wrestler's skin seems to become remarkably resistant to mat burns; a karate expert's hand can be used like a hatchet to break a board; and even one's crotch and seat quickly adapt themselves to saddle trauma after a few days of horseback riding. Blisters are replaced by calluses, strained muscles relax, and discomforts disappear as the body adapts itself to new demands. Commonplace observations of this kind increase my respect for the dynamic potentialities of the human central nervous system, which is constantly striving to keep in tune with the demands of both its internal and external environment. And when anything acts to throw it off stride, either mental or physical, nothing seems more likely to restore normal function than the establishment of a normal input.

14

Peripheral and Central Mechanisms of Causalgia

I would naturally prefer to talk about my surgical successes rather than my failures, but often a case that does not go according to expectations teaches you more than one that goes smoothly. One of the most difficult cases that I have ever been called upon to treat was Mr. C.S., a 35-year-old mill worker who suffered from a severe ulnar causalgia of long standing. I treated this patient several years before the young man (Lee) described in the previous chapter.[1] On November 25, 1935, C.S. had been working near some heavy machinery when a belt broke, striking him and throwing him against a timber. His right humerus was fractured transversely at the junction of its upper and middle thirds. Ever since this accident he had complained bitterly of pain. An aching pain in his upper arm extended into his axilla, chest, and neck, and he felt a terrible burning sensation in his hand. The ring and little fingers felt "numb" and "half asleep," yet were exquisitely sensitive to touch. Several times each day the forearm muscles would "go into a cramp," so that the fingers, particularly the ring and little fingers, were drawn tightly into his palm and he "had to work them loose" with the other hand. He noted that these two fingers were constantly cold, discolored, and wet with sweat.

I first examined this man for the Industrial Accident Commission early in 1938. His fractured humerus had never united despite four

---

[1]*Editor's Note:* Livingston described this same patient (C.S.) in his 1943 book. In this chapter he is more focused on the possibility of antidromic release of pain-producing substances as postulated by Lewis.

operations on the bone. The first "sliding graft" had absorbed soon after it was put into place. Twice the Boehler procedure of boring a hole into the callus ends had been tried and then a large graft was taken from his tibia but this, too, had disappeared. Some fibrous union had occurred, but any movement at the fracture site or any pressure on the arm near it aggravated his pains intolerably. The man looked thin and pain-worn and had lost twenty-two pounds since his accident. He was surly and uncooperative and had developed a deep resentment toward all physicians because they seemed to be interested only in the non-union and not in his pain. He said that he "didn't give a damn about the fracture" but he *had* to have relief from "the terrible burning pain." He claimed, "My whole right side seems to be affected; my right eye blurs when I try to read; my chest and neck on that side hurt most of the time and my right leg is weak and often gives way under me."

During my examination he kept his hand carefully guarded from any contact and was reluctant to have it examined. The ring and little finger, particularly the distal two joints of the ring finger, were red and shiny and the nails were opaque and long. He dared not cut these two fingernails because it so aggravated his pain, but at times they were accidentally broken off. The ulnar side of the hand was glistening wet with perspiration and when he hung the hand down the drops of sweat fell from the end of the ring finger every few seconds. Despite the subjective sensation of burning, the right hand was colder than the left; the ring and little finger measured 2°C colder than the same fingers of the left hand. At the level of the ununited fracture there was a palpable enlargement of the ulnar nerve trunk that was extremely sensitive to pressure. The injection of procaine solution into the nerve trunk above this fusiform enlargement relieved his pain for several hours. Two other methods could confer temporary relief. One was to block this upper dorsal sympathetic chain on the right; the other was to block the ulnar nerve near the elbow. The latter is of interest because the injection was several inches *distal* to the irritative nerve lesion.

On May 18, 1938, exposure of the ulnar nerve in the upper arm revealed it to be partially divided with a laterally protruding mass of fibers embedded in the highly vascular scar tissue. The damaged segment of nerve was excised and an end-to-end anastomosis performed. The relief from pain was complete and immediate, and the change in the patient was dramatic. Instead of a disgruntled and antisocial patient lying in a bed for hours with his face to the wall, he was up and about the hospital ward, chatting cheerfully with the nurses and the patients. He left the hospital convinced that his suffering was over and planned to return soon for another operation on the bone. After two months the pain began to recur and by October it was as bad as ever. Between November 1938 and the following April, a series of procaine injections successfully blocked the ulnar nerve above the anastomosis, the brachial plexus, and the stellate ganglion. Each procedure gave him considerable relief that tended to outlast the local effects of the procaine but never persisted for more than a week. A second resection of the nerve and a new anastomosis not only failed to relieve the pain but seemed to aggravate all his symptoms. Thereafter, a combination of stellate ganglion blocks and an injection of the anastomotic area were sufficient to hold his pain under reasonable control until early in 1940. Then the effectiveness of both these procedures tended to diminish and a stellate block on February 13, 1940, increased the intensity of his suffering immediately after the injection, while the Horner's syndrome was still evident.

In July 1940 I performed a third resection of the nerve trunk. It was necessary to transpose the ulnar trunk at the elbow to obtain sufficient length to anastomose the cut ends. Given the failure of the second resection to relieve his symptoms, neither the patient nor I expected too much benefit from the third resection, but we were delighted by the immediate and complete pain relief. In September he reported a weight gain of twelve pounds and was sleeping and eating well. He felt less local sensitivity in the operative area than at any previous time. He remained quite comfortable until the middle of October when he caught a cold and coughing spells brought back the pain in his chest, axilla, and upper arm. Within a few weeks the pain was again as bad as ever, with the whole right side affected. He refused to permit any treatment to the bone until his pain had been controlled. He urged me to try another nerve resection. I told him that if I cut out any more of the nerve trunk it would be impossible to ever again unite the cut ends. He said that he didn't care about the function of his hand and would gladly let me cut the arm off if only I could assure him that this would end his suffering. I finally consented to permanently sacrifice the ulnar nerve in the belief that perhaps if I could get it high above the old area of injury and left the cut end well out of the scar tissue, the source of irritation would be gone. This was done but only partially relieved his pain, which gradually returned to full force.

Before resorting to a high chordotomy or a posterior rhizotomy, I made two more attempts to secure a bony union at the fracture site on the theory that irritation caused by slight movement there might be keeping the pain process active. The first attempt failed when the patient claimed that his cast made the pain intolerable and so tore it off. The second procedure consisted of a "step operation" and this time the patient was kept in the hospital and given large doses of analgesia and hypnotic drugs until it was apparent that a solid union would occur. After his operation I attributed the gradual fading of his complaints to the sedative drugs, but his improvement persisted after all medication stopped. In 1942 he was sufficiently improved to permit his claim against the Accident Commission to be closed with a partial disability rating.

I am not proud of my handling of this case. Looking back on it from the vantage point of our present knowledge of causalgia, I think that the whole tragic sequence might have been averted or at least shortened by different treatment. A sympathectomy in which the second, third, and fourth thoracic ganglia were removed on the left side might have stopped his pain, particularly if it had been done early, before the process had gained too much headway. It seems likely that if the lesion of the ulnar nerve had been recognized sooner after the accident, a resection and anastomosis might have relieved his symptoms and perhaps ensured a survival of the bone graft. It is possible that if I had done something to secure a solid union at the fracture site during the first resection, more than two years after his accident, that his pain would not have recurred. In suggesting these alternatives, I am not apologizing for the treatment I gave this patient. I developed a very real affection for this man during our long association and would have gone to any lengths to help him. However, as I see it now, my fault was focusing too much attention on the local nerve lesion. My treatment was a sort of "hand-to-mouth" affair in which I was successful in relieving his symptoms for short periods by removing most of the sources of irritation but never quite enough to permit the central process to subside permanently. I should have seen more clearly the possible significance of two observations: that a sympathetic block relieved his symptoms, as did a block of the ulnar nerve *distal* to the lesion.

Later, after more experience with causalgic states, I gave even more attention to the possible implications of these two observations. I shall discuss them in subsequent chapters but for now I am concerned only with one: that a procaine block distal to the lesion temporarily stopped this patient's pain. I cannot recall why I tried this injection; perhaps only so I could examine his sensitive hand more carefully. I do remember that the patient and I reacted differently to the result. From his point of view the pain was originating in his sensitive hand. It was a logical assumption that a block that numbed the hand should stop his pain. From my viewpoint, the relief afforded by the injection was not logical at all. I had decided that the pain was a psychological process in the man's brain and merely "projected" by him to the hand. I visualized the source of irritation in the local lesion in the ulnar nerve near the fracture site. Since the procaine was not interposed between this source and the brain, it did not seem logical that the injection should alter the pain as it obviously did nor that the pain relief should persist after the local anesthetic effects had worn off. Since I could not deny the clinical evidence, it must be that my logic had proceeded from a false premise. Apparently I was wrong in assuming that the whole story of "causalgia" was to be found in the local nerve lesion. The lesion certainly started the syndrome but other factors must develop secondarily, either at the periphery or within the central nervous system, to account for the "build-up" and "spread" of signs and symptoms.

One possible explanation for the relief of pain after an injection of procaine distal to the lesion was that the true source of the irritation to the sensory nerves was not in the lesion itself but in the tissues within its peripheral distribution. Perhaps the nerve lesion stimulated motor fibers or created antidromic impulses in the sensory fibers that led to the elaboration of some chemical irritant that gave rise to pain and the local hyperalgesia. Perhaps C.S. was right in thinking that the local sensitivity and pain were originating in the hand itself. If true, a nerve block at the elbow would temporarily abolish them. However, how could I account for the burning pain ascribed to the hand after the nerve had been resected?

A second possible explanation might be that the nerve lesion acted something like a "voltage booster" on a transmission line. Perhaps it "boosted" all incoming impulse patterns above the pain threshold. If this were so, a distal block would stop the sensory input and leave little or nothing to "boost," thus relieving the pain.

There was still another possible explanation. Perhaps the nerve lesion constantly assaulted the central nervous system with a barrage of afferent impulses of abnormal intensity until its normal activities were seriously deranged. Perhaps this central sensitization resulted in a shunting of all incoming messages into the pain pathways. Was there any evidence to support the concept of a "central excitatory state"? At what level did it develop? Did it involve the internuncial pool in the spinal cord at the level of the first sensory relay, the thalamus, or the "sensorium," or perhaps all three levels together?

I do not mean to imply that I was doing any such tight reasoning at the time I was treating C.S. All I knew then was that my preconceived notions about the mechanisms underlying the syndrome of causalgia were incomplete at best. I was in a state of confusion and groping blindly for any explanation that might fit the facts better. I remember how excited I was when I first read Sir Thomas Lewis's studies of hyperalgesia in which he postulated the existence of "nocifensor" neurons. Here was proof that irritation of the sensory nerve led to the elaboration of a chemical irritant in the peripheral tissues that could account for the hyperalgesia that was so prominent a feature of causalgia, and might explain why a nerve block distal to a lesion could relieve pain.

Hyperalgesia

The easiest way to produce cutaneous hyperalgesia experimentally is to pick up a bit of skin in a toothed forceps and give it a strong pinch. Within a few minutes the surrounding skin shows an altered sensibility in which the innocuous stimuli give rise to unpleasant or painful sensations. The zone of hyperalgesia may spread distally for considerable distances and its extent is roughly proportional to the severity of the crushing injury inflicted by the forceps. Gellhorn and colleagues (1931) studied hyperalgesia and concluded that the intensification, unpleasantness, and indefinite local signs that characterize sensory responses to stimulation are due to a disturbance of activity in the spinal cord, phenomena he referred to as "spinal radiation." Dusser de Barenne (1931) demonstrated that hyperalgesia can be induced peripherally by injecting small amounts of strychnine into the posterior horns of gray matter of the spinal cord. Echlin and Propper (1937) showed that a preliminary scraping of a frog's skin increased the frequency of nerve impulses conducted along sensory nerves as a result of simple pressure stimuli. They believed that the scraping produced a change in the skin that "hypersensitized" it and altered the sensory responses to innocuous stimuli.

In 1937 Sir Thomas Lewis published his extensive studies of cutaneous hyperalgesia (Lewis 1939, 1942). He found that if the skin is first infiltrated with procaine, the experimental crushing is rendered painless and no hyperalgesia develops in the surrounding skin until the local anesthesia has disappeared. He could produce a spreading hyperalgesia by directly stimulating a sensory nerve branch, but a procaine block proximal to the point of stimulation delayed hyperalgesia until the nerve fibers regained their conductivity. If he blocked conduction in the fibers distal to the point of stimulation the skin became hyperalgesic around the site of the stimulation but it did not progress distally beyond the procaine block until the local anesthetic effect had disappeared. These and other experiments conducted by Lewis demonstrated two important facts: cutaneous hyperalgesia is due, at least in part, to the elaboration of some chemical substance in the skin, and the process is mediated by sensory nerves.

15

Procaine and Nitrous Oxide "Analgesia"

After completing my surgical internship before beginning private practice I served for two years as director of the Student Health Service at the University of Oregon in Eugene. During this interval my interest in visceral pain problems remained as active as ever in regard to my reading, but I performed so few major surgical operations that my opportunities to make direct observations of visceral sensibility were limited. The nature of my assignment forced me to temporarily shift my attention to the somatic pains arising from injuries to muscles, bones, and joints. In caring for this type of injury, I sometimes found myself in competition with nonmedical trainers and coaches whose rough-and-ready methods for treating accidental injuries often seemed unjustifiable. The particular form of treatment that offended me most was their habit of treating acute injuries by the injection of procaine solutions (then called "novocaine") into injured muscles or around damaged joints to relieve the man's pain during a competitive game and permit him to immediately resume play. It seemed to me that coaches were so anxious to win athletic contests they were disregarding the best interests of the injured man. My instinct was to put such a man to bed and apply hot, moist packs to the injured part. I had been taught that tissue injury plus pain were indications for complete rest of the injured limb and protection from further injury. I felt I ought to put a stop to the promiscuous use of procaine injections.

One day, a key man on the varsity basketball team came to my office complaining of a painful right foot. The man could not recall having injured this foot at any time, but for several days it had been getting increasingly sensitive over the lateral aspect and now the pain was so severe that he no longer could work out with the team. His foot was tender to pressure over the fifth metatarsal bone but there was no swelling or discoloration in this area and an X-ray picture failed to show any detectable abnormality in the bones or joints. After a few days in bed with hot packs on his foot, this man complained that the foot hurt him worse than ever if he tried to put any weight on it. A second X-ray showed an oblique, linear fracture of the fifth metatarsal bone in its middle third. About this time the basketball coach came to see me to ask when I would let the player return to team practice. He looked at the X-ray picture and advised me to inject procaine solution around the fracture site and then get the man back on his feet. He said, "That fracture will never heal under the treatment you are giving him!" I was equally certain that the treatment the coach suggested would make the condition worse.

After a few more days of bed rest, there being no signs of improvement, I compromised by applying a walking cast on the injured foot and allowing the patient to get out of bed and walk with the assistance of crutches. The cast was bivalved to permit physiotherapy treatments each day. After a few weeks a third X-ray picture of the foot showed that the fracture line was much wider than previously and the metatarsal bone showed a diffuse, spotty loss of density with no evidence of any callus formation. At the end of ten weeks the man reported the foot was more painful then ever, and a fourth X-ray film revealed that all the bones of the foot now showed a marked loss of density and a diffuse osteoporosis. This picture really scared me because the bones looked like Swiss cheese that had been gnawed on by rats. In a chastened spirit I began daily injections of procaine around the fracture site and followed each with active manipulation of the badly stiffened foot and full weight bearing as long as the analgesic effect of the injection persisted. Under this new regime the sensitivity, swelling, and stiffness rapidly decreased and within ten days a fifth X-ray picture showed definite evidence of a beginning callus formation. Recovery was rapid from then on, although not until several weeks after this man began playing basketball again did the bones of the foot regain their normal density.

This was my first introduction to the peculiar pain states that occasionally follow trauma to bones and joints and which are referred to as "traumatic osteoporosis," "reflex dystrophy," and "Sudeck's atrophy."

They are characterized by severe pain that seems way out of proportion to the degree of the injury and there are often signs of vasomotor and sudomotor disturbances in the affected part before a spreading osteoporosis becomes visible in an X-ray film. No one knows what causes these bizarre pain syndromes and this is not the place to speculate as to their possible underlying mechanisms. Instead, I wish to relate another incident involving the use of procaine injections to deaden pain after acute trauma, followed by the immediate resumption of normal use of the part. This incident occurred a few years after I had started private practice in Portland, Oregon. The physician who had taken my place in the University Student Health Service was a man whom I liked and whose judgment I respected. He accompanied the University of Oregon football team when they came to Portland to play a game against the University of Washington in Multnomah Stadium. This physician invited me to sit with him on the team bench during the game.

During the second quarter of the game Oregon's star quarterback sustained such a painful injury to his right thigh that he had to be carried off the field. During the intermission I went to the locker rooms to see how badly he had been injured and what treatment my physician friend was giving him. The player's thigh was swollen and hard to palpation as if a massive hemorrhage had occurred deep within the quadriceps muscle. The thigh was so stiff and painful that the man could neither bend his knee nor bear weight on the leg. The physician used a large syringe and a long needle to inject procaine solution throughout the injured muscle mass. As soon as the injection had produced its analgesic effect the man got off the table and walked around the room. The muscle spasm seemed to have disappeared and he insisted he could use the leg as well as ever. He returned to the game and played the entire second half without showing any evidence of disability. I watched him closely to see if he favored the injured limb, as I expected he would after the procaine effects had worn off, but as far as I could tell he played with all his usual speed and skill. Subsequently, I talked with both the man and his physician about this form of treatment and they both insisted that it did no harm and they were inclined to think that it had hastened his recovery. Whether or not a return to scrimmage, with its danger of further damage to the injured muscle, was in the best interests of this athlete is not the main issue here. I am only calling attention to the fact that the short-lasting, analgesic effect of the procaine seemed to restore a completely disabled player to full efficiency for a surprisingly long time.

These and other similar observations were making me less cocky and less rigid in my ideas as to how to treat acute injuries attended by disabling degrees of pain. I began to use procaine injections in the treatment of acute sprains, followed by supportive strapping with adhesive tape and active use of the limb. I found that similar injections, carefully localized in tender spots and followed by deep massage and exercise, were often successful in relieving such conditions as "tennis elbow," "charley horse," and "subdeltoid bursitis." Sometimes the relief of pain and the immediate restoration of free movement were described by the patient as "miraculous." I did not think it was miraculous because I had expected that the relief of pain would relax the muscle spasm that was limiting movement and adding to the pain.

But what did seem to me miraculous was that in many such instances the relief was permanent. Sometimes the injections failed to relieve all the pain or several injections might be needed before recovery was established, but I had the impression that when the injection was made in exactly the right spot, the whole symptom complex would melt away. Why this happened I did not know, but I began to search for "trigger points" that might be the source of some complex reflex process that was sustaining the pain and disability. And I was beginning to wonder if a peripheral source of chronic irritation might not be able to create some disturbance of function within the spinal cord in much the same way that Ross, Head, and MacKenzie had imagined that abnormal input from an internal organ could set up a central disturbance that might create "referred phenomena."

While these speculations were beginning to take vague form I was also becoming greatly interested in the analgesia produced by the inhalation of small amounts of ether or nitrous oxide and oxygen. As every medical student knows, during the induction of a state of general anesthesia produced by these drugs, the patient passes through a series of "stages" before he goes deeply asleep and his muscles relax. The first of these stages is called the "stage of analgesia" because in it the patient loses much or all of his ability to feel painful stimuli before his other perceptual faculties become seriously impaired. During the two years I headed the Student Health Service, physicians in many parts of the country were making efforts to control this transient stage of analgesia while they carried out minor surgical operations. Manufacturers of gas oxygen machines were becoming interested in these efforts and had put "dots" on the dials of their machines to indicate the exact proportions of nitrous oxide and oxygen that should produce the desired state of "analgesia." I was aware of this interesting line of investigation when I first came to the Health Service and I wanted to have a part in it. One of my first requests to the authorities was permission to purchase a particular gas-oxygen machine that I knew had these "dots" on the mixing gauge dial. I told the authorities that we needed this machine for the clinic because we have to do so many minor surgical operations, some of which precluded the use of procaine analgesia, and the only alternative we had to offer was ether anesthesia. I explained that nitrous oxide was much more pleasant to take than ether, and that its effects were of shorter duration and less messy. These persuasive arguments had the desired effect and in due time a Heidbrink gas-oxygen machine arrived in a huge crate. With it came two enormous tanks, one filled with nitrous oxide, the other with oxygen.

These deliveries were made at the Health Service offices on a Saturday afternoon when all my assistants had left for the day. I uncrated the machine and connected it to the gas tanks. Once it seemed in good working order I could not resist the temptation to try a few simple experiments on myself. I adjusted the gas flow from the two tanks until the gauge showed delivery of exactly the right amount of each drug that should be expected to produce a state of analgesia. I laid a sharp scalpel on the window ledge where I could easily reach it while sitting in my swivel office chair. I settled comfortably in the chair and breathed in the gas mixture while holding the mask against my face. When I thought I must have reached the stage of analgesia I laid aside the mask, picked up the knife, and made a small cut on my left hand with it. This test was not conclusive. Although the pain caused by the cutting may well have been partially dulled, I certainly felt pain when I made any sizable cut. I thought that perhaps this could be explained by the need to lay aside the mask while doing the cutting.

Perhaps I was analgesic while the mask was in place and I was breathing the gas, but this state might rapidly disappear when I took a few breaths of room air. I then tried biting one of my hands to test for pain sensation because I only needed to tip the mask slightly in order to bite myself. I still felt pain if I bit hard, so I rummaged around in the accessory kit and found a small mask that fitted nicely over my nose while leaving my mouth exposed. I could also use both hands because the mask was held in place by an elastic band around my head.

With the nasal mask on I carried out more tests. I was convinced that the gas mixture definitely dulled my pain sensibility but it never completely abolished it. I decided that perhaps the percentage of nitrous oxide was not high enough to induce full analgesia for a man of my large size and weight. I sweetened the mixture and picked up the knife. As I went on breathing the gas I seemed to forget what I was supposed to be doing, for I laid aside the knife and just sat staring at the machine for a time. I recall thinking what a pretty machine it was and how brightly its metal and glassware sparkled. I had a vague notion that I ought to turn the thing off, but I was not particularly concerned when I found I was unable to reach the control valves. That was the last thing I can remember. I awoke after an indefinite period of time to find myself lying on my side on the office floor. There was a puddle of saliva under my head where I had drooled during my sleep. The mask was still in place and it was some time before I could remember why I was wearing it and how I happened to fall asleep sprawled out on the floor. As I became better oriented I could tell that the machine was still running because I could hear the sustained hiss of the escaping gases. When I removed the mask and sat up, I saw that the large flexible tube leading from the machine to the mask had become disconnected at the gas outlet. Evidently in falling from my chair I had jerked the tube from its connection to the machine.

The swivel chair in which I had been sitting was one in which I could tilt back comfortably in a stable position but, fortunately, in this instance I must have been sitting forward in the chair, perhaps in an effort to reach the control valves, so that I fell forward instead of backward. They were large tanks.

That was my last solo effort in experimenting with nitrous oxide analgesia and one I was careful not to mention at home for a long time. In all subsequent experiments I worked with the physician who was next in command at the Health Service. We carried out many experiments on each other and on a few students who consented to serve as test subjects. We also performed a number of minor surgical procedures using this technique. We agreed that after a few breaths of the gas mixture the subject's ability to feel pain was definitely diminished. If the dosage was just right for a particular test subject, his ability to feel pain was lost before his vision, hearing, or his ability to talk or move voluntarily became seriously impaired. It was our impression that the perception of pain was being selectively suppressed rather than that the pain had been experienced and subsequently forgotten. We were able to lance boils and do other minor operations under this form of analgesia provided these procedures could be carried out rapidly and at exactly the right moment. Our principal difficulty was our inability to hold the subject in a satisfactory state of analgesia for any length of time. The stage of analgesia evidently represented a very narrow zone between full consciousness and the next lower "stage of excitement." In this second stage the subject is neither fully asleep nor fully awake, but he is mentally confused and his behavior often resembles that of an alcoholic in a fighting jag. He tends to talk incoherently or to laugh immoderately (hence the former name for nitrous oxide, "laughing gas") and he reacts violently to any noxious stimulus even though he may later say that he felt no pain at any time. His physical response to any harmful stimulus tends to be so completely unrestrained that his efforts to fight back or escape may result in injury to himself or his attendants.

The excitement stage induced by nitrous oxide gas was of great interest to me, although it was difficult to make its implications fit with my pattern of the push-button concept of pain. I had always thought that the pattern of impulses set up by a noxious stimulus was carried by the specific pain fiber into the spinal cord to do two things in quick succession: first it set off a train of involuntary reflex responses in the body and then it ascended the pain and temperature tract to the brain where it registered as pain. I believed that both parts of the defensive mechanism were directly dependent upon stimulus intensity. In fact, I had been told that pain could be measured in terms of stimulus intensity. Based on this belief, physiologists had transferred their study of pain from human subjects to experimental animals. Yet our observations of subjects in the excitement stage produced by nitrous oxide inhalations suggested that pain perception was depressed while body reflex responses were increasing as if all brakes had been removed from their expression. The implication seemed to be that both these effects of the drug were acting on the nervous system above the point at which the central ends of pain fibers terminated in the spinal cord.

Based on what my assistant and I had learned about the site of action of anesthetic drugs, we could assume that both effects of nitrous oxide administration must involve cortical cells. Nerve cells in the cerebral cortex were supposed to be more susceptible to the action of drugs than were cells in any other part of the central nervous system. Because the control of voluntary movement was also assumed to originate in cortical cells, we could assume that the action of the nitrous oxide would result in both the suppression of pain and the release of the reflex mechanisms from voluntary control.

My assistant and I spent a good deal of time discussing interpretations of this kind because, in the two years of our association in the Health Service, he had become as much interested in pain problems as I was. From our study of nitrous oxide analgesia we had drawn three general conclusions: (1) This method for controlling pain will never be of much practical importance to surgeons; (2) Pain is *not* measurable in terms of the body reflex responses to noxious stimuli. Our arguments also involved a third conclusion that we reached triumphantly: (3) Pain is a *specific* sensation. I was inclined to question the specificity of the pain fiber, and from what I had read about the results of chordotomies for the relief of pain, I doubted that the anterolateral spinothalamic tract was the only route by which pain sensation could reach a perceptual level. He felt that my doubts were ill-founded and maintained that our observations of the state of analgesia provided final proof that the three-neuron pain pathway was specific from end to end. His argument started with the assumption that pain perception is a function of nerve cells in the cerebral cortex. Such calls *must* be specific for pain because, when a person inhales nitrous oxide gas, the ability to perceive pain is lost before other sensory perceptions are seriously impaired. Thus, the cortical cells subserving pain perception must be different from those subserving other sensory perceptions. The ability of the person to localize the source of pain and evaluate its qualities must mean that the pain pathway represents a point-to-point route from the site of stimulation to these specialized cortical cells.

In closing this chapter I must again admit that I am drawing on my imagination in trying to reconstitute interpretations made so many years ago, although I am confident that their general import is reasonably accurate. I must also admit that most of the conclusions reached at that time were later proven wrong. To illustrate this point, I will mention only one conclusion that my assistant and I reached after our study of nitrous oxide analgesia. We were convinced that it would never be possible to carry out surgical procedures of any duration while maintaining the patient in an analgesic state. This conclusion seemed reasonable enough based on our observations, but it was wrong. Let me describe an operation under "analgesia" as it is carried out in a modern hospital.

A woman is lying on an operating table while a surgeon is repairing one of her heart valves. Her eyes are open and she is apparently aware of what the anesthesiologist is saying to her. At the moment he is asking her how many children she has. She is unable to reply directly because she has a tracheal tube protruding from her mouth but she can nod or shake her head when he mentions a particular number or holds up the appropriate number of fingers. "One?"—a vigorous shake of her head. "Ten?"—a stronger shake of the head and a grimace. "Three?"—and she happily nods her head in affirmation. All this while the surgeon is cutting and sewing on her heart and chest wall. She is evidently able to see, hear, think, and move voluntarily but she gives no evidence that the surgical procedures are causing her any pain. The operation may go on for an hour or more and for all this time the patient remains in a satisfactory state of analgesia.

What has the anesthesiologist done that we did not do and that results in this prolonged state of analgesia? He had used a mixture of oxygen and some anesthetic gas just as we had, but instead of trying to maintain the patient in the early "stage of analgesia" he had administered enough of the mixture to put her deeply asleep before the operation began. Then, as the operation proceeded, he gradually lightened the depth of the anesthetic state until the patient entered the state of analgesia "through the back door," so to speak.

It is easier to describe this trick that the anesthesiologist employs to achieve a state of analgesia than it is to explain why it is successful. This problem will be discussed in later chapters and all that needs to be said about it here is that over the years scientists have been learning more about how and where anesthetic drugs act on the central nervous system. This new knowledge is giving them quite a different picture of how a brain may carry out its complex functions than I have suggested in this chapter.

16

Hypnosis

I have often been asked if I think that hypnosis has any legitimate place in the practice of surgery, obstetrics, or dentistry. I have never known how to answer this question, particularly when asked by some young surgeon on the staff. I was aware that it had become something of a fad among young practitioners to try their hand at hypnotizing patients. I could not approve the promiscuous use of hypnosis by untrained persons any more than I could approve the promiscuous use of trance-inducing drugs by amateur psychiatrists. Yet, I have seen enough to convince me that in skilled hands hypnosis holds some strange influence over body functions and pain perceptions. Until medical science can offer better evidence as to where and how hypnosis can alter function in the human nervous system, its legitimate place among our therapeutic tools must remain in doubt. In seeking such information I would hope that scientists would try to approach the problem with an open mind. However, having said that I have been convinced that hypnosis can exert an influence on pain perception, the subject becomes part of my story that I ought not to sidestep simply because I am on unfamiliar ground in an area strongly colored by prejudice.

Several years ago, a member of my surgical staff showed me the chart of a woman a week after she had had plastic surgery on her neck. I already was familiar with this woman's history. As a child she had suffered an extensive burn of her face, neck, and chest. She had been left with a massive scar that was pulling her chin down to her chest. To free her head and neck movements, she had been undergoing a series of operations and she had been on our surgical wards on several occasions.

During these admissions she had disturbed all the patients in her vicinity with her loud and persistent complaints of pain after each operation. These complaints had persisted throughout her hospital stay despite the administration of considerable amounts of opiates and other analgesic drugs. However, her behavior had been quite different during her present admission. The chart showed that her postoperative course had been unusually smooth. She had made few complaints of pain and had been given only one dose of a half grain of codeine the first day after surgery. When I asked why her behavior had changed in this striking fashion I was told that the plastic surgeon who had done the last operation was Dr. S., who had controlled her pain with hypnosis. I had known that Dr. S. used hypnosis in caring for patients in his private practice and I had been told that on a few occasions he had used it successfully in carrying out surgical operations in our University Hospital. I had been skeptical about this report. I had always associated hypnosis with stage shows and quackery. Yet, the evidence in this case suggested that I might be letting my prejudices blind me to something I ought to know more about. Also, I was curious as to what Dr. S. knew about hypnosis and how he had got started using it in his practice.

In subsequent talks with Dr. S. I learned that he had begun to practice various methods for inducing hypnotic states when he was quite young. His mother had been a wardrobe mistress in a Vienna theater and S. had seen many demonstrations of hypnosis on the stage. Since obtaining his medical degree and training in plastic surgery, he had used hypnosis on many occasions and had found it to be a useful adjunct in his surgical work. In his opinion there was nothing mysterious about hypnosis; it was merely a powerful form of "suggestion." While he had found certain patients to be particularly susceptible to suggestion therapy of this kind, he believed that every normal person was susceptible to it in some degree. He felt that this influence was not only exerted by physicians intentionally but was constantly being exerted by all physicians, nurses, members of the family, and even casual visitors. The sincere sympathy and ministrations to the patient's needs by attendants were all a part of this form of therapy and could alleviate suffering. He was convinced that the practice of hypnosis had been used consciously or unconsciously by priests and medicine men from prehistoric times. To illustrate this point he described the itinerant "tooth-pullers" he had watched as a child in Armenia.

The equipment of such a tooth-puller was simple. It consisted of faggots[1] with which to build a fire, a piece of strap iron to heat in the flame, and several sheets of heavy wrapping paper that could be laid against the patient's swollen jaw while the hot iron was rubbed gently over it. The equipment might also contain one or two pairs of pliers, although these men had so much strength in their finger grip that they rarely had to resort to pliers to remove abscessed teeth. Suppose now that a tooth-puller is approached by a man with an abscessed tooth and a jaw so swollen that he is unable to open his mouth. The two men find a place beside the road where they can sit comfortably side by side, while the tooth-puller builds his little fire and starts the iron heating. All the time he is sympathizing with the patient, rubbing his back, and assuring him that he will feel no pain during the extraction and that once the tooth is out, all his troubles will be over. When the iron is quite hot but not enough to singe the paper, a few layers of paper are held against the jaw while the iron is rubbed over them. Under the influence of the heat and the encouragement, the jaw muscles relax until the patient can open his mouth so that the tooth-puller can see the offending tooth. Then with an arm over the patient's shoulders and still talking, he reaches in and jerks out the tooth. The patient spits a few times, assures all within hearing distance that he felt no pain, adds his thanks to the small fee charged for the extraction, and goes happily on his way.

I asked Dr. S. if he would be willing to demonstrate the usefulness of hypnosis in controlling pain before one of my classes of medical students. He consented and on the appointed day I found that he had brought to the classroom four of his patients, three children in wheelchairs and the woman with the scar contractures whose chart I had seen. She had been wheeled in from the ward in her bed. In my opening remarks to the students I said that this demonstration did not imply any particular attitude on my part toward the use of hypnosis to control pain. I also reminded them that a classroom full of students was not an ideal place in which to conduct a test of this kind and that, like children called upon to perform for company, these patients might not respond well to hypnotic suggestions. Dr. S. started his demonstration with the woman in bed. She had been lying quietly listening to my

---

[1]A bundle of sticks or twigs bound together for fuel.

remarks and looking over the assembled students with an expression of mild interest. After talking to her a while, Dr. S. exposed her right forearm, rubbed it with some alcohol, and draped some sterile towels around it, meantime explaining to the patient that he was going to put a few surgical sutures in the skin of her forearm but that she would feel no pain and the temporary presence of the sutures would do her no harm. Then he donned a pair of sterile gloves and used a cutting needle and coarse dermol suture material to put in a row of sutures. I was standing by the bed but could detect no sign that the woman felt any discomfort while the sutures were being inserted.

Then, to my surprise, Dr. S. said to her: "All right, now you can wake up." She gave a quick start, fluttered her eyelids, excitedly looked around the room, and demanded to know who all these people were and what had been happening. Then she noticed the sutures in her forearm and asked who put them there and for what purpose. She quieted down when Dr. S. reminded her that he had previously told her the purpose of the class demonstration and her part in it and that she had freely given her consent to take part. He then explained to the students that what I had said about a classroom being a poor place in which to induce a hypnotic state was correct. Knowing this, he had taken the precaution to hypnotize all four patients before bringing them to the classroom.

The physician from whom I learned the most about hypnosis was Dr. Ainslie Meares, a psychiatrist in Melbourne, Australia, who had won worldwide fame for his skillful use of this therapeutic agency. He rather reluctantly permitted me to make a few simple tests of pain perception on some of his patients while he used hypnosis to treat their various physical and mental complaints. The tests were made only on patients who gave their consent and while they were in a relatively light state of hypnosis so that they could report their subjective sensory experiences during the tests. The stimuli used consisted largely of pricking, pinching, or pressing deeply on the skin of one arm while this limb was in normal or abnormal postures. It was interesting that none of the patients seemed to have any difficulty in localizing the source of the stimulus and its nature except that they invariably denied that the evoked sensation was painful. They usually knew whether I was using the head or the point of a pin to press on the skin and they might even use the words "sharp" and "dull" to describe their subjective experience, yet they either ignored or did not feel pain even when the skin penetration was sudden and deep, nor did they exhibit any withdrawal reactions. Muscular relaxation was constantly maintained and they made no effort to correct abnormal postures that would soon be distressing under normal circumstances. Dr. Meares commented that when he put a patient into a deep hypnotic sleep at the end of each treatment he checked to see that the patient's posture was comfortable because patients never spontaneously corrected abnormal postures or pressures. He seemed to think that the danger of muscle strain, pressure sores, or nerve paralyses was as great for a patient in a hypnotic sleep as for patients under general anesthesia.

The test Dr. Meares performed with me as a subject was conducted in the presence of two neurosurgeons during a private session in his home library. I willingly consented to let him hypnotize me while I was sitting in a large leather armchair with my arms extended comfortably on the padded chair arms. He began by asking me to close my eyes while he moved my right forearm back and forth, as my elbow rested on the chair arm. In the meantime he talked quietly to me and made his customary suggestions to "relax" each part of my body, each part becoming heavier and heavier, even my eyelids becoming so heavy that I could not open my eyes, etc., etc., etc. He then let go of my arm while suggesting that the movement would continue automatically. I continued to move the arm but it was my impression that I was doing it voluntarily just to please Dr. Meares. I did not think that I was hypnotized but he evidently thought so. He laid my arm down in a restful position and made a deep cut in the skin of my forearm with a razor blade. The cut was about one and a half inches long, drew blood, and evidently penetrated all the skin layers because it left a permanent scar. I definitely felt pain during the cutting, although the observers said I made no overt response and my pulse rate did not change. Then I was told to wake up and while the wound was being dressed I was asked if I had felt any pain. I said that I had, and added that I doubted that I had been hypnotized. The others insisted that I must have been, otherwise I would have shown more response to the cutting.

I told them that for many years I had practiced Jacobsen's "art of progressive relaxation" and had found that the ability to relax muscles in all parts of the body not only helped me to get to sleep after I had been under some emotional strain but it also enabled me to tolerate more pain than when in any other body state. They were skeptical about this until I showed them some of the scars I had received while voluntarily holding my arm against the aperture of the "dolorimeter" while the heat was creating a deep burn. My friends seemed to doubt my claims, so I said, "All right, you all agree that I am not now hypnotized. Give me a few minutes to relax and then one of you can make an equally deep cut in the skin of my left forearm, while you watch to see if I make any more reactions to the cutting than when I was 'hypnotized.'" An equally deep cut was then made on my left forearm (also leaving a permanent scar) but they could observe no visible response as the razor blade was dragged slowly though the skin. Nor did I think there was any essential difference in my subjective experiences during the two experiments.

Of course, experiments of this kind are not well enough controlled to prove anything. They merely suggest that various body states, including muscular relaxation and physical exhaustion as well as hypnotic states, seem to dull pain perception. But I doubt that pain perception is dependent upon neural processes involving a single channel that can be turned on or off like water at a faucet. I have many reasons for thinking that pain relief, no matter how it is induced, is always dependent upon an interaction between many neural forces and is usually *relative* rather than absolute. I want to mention four observations that seem to support this opinion because they may indicate why I think that hypnosis must involve some general neural mechanism that we ordinarily associate with suggestion or some atavistic reversion to a more primitive mental level.

I made the first observation while I was examining a method two Australian investigators were using to evaluate the analgesic potency of new drugs. They had devised some ingenious ways to record the minimal amount of pressure on a dog's ear or the strength of an electrical shock to its leg just sufficient to elicit a response (i.e., the threshold) in a normal dog. Then they determined what influence a particular drug had in raising this threshold. As a "baseline" they had recorded the dog's threshold after a massive dose of morphine, and then they expressed the analgesic potency of the new drug as a percentage of the maximum morphine effect. I asked these lads if they thought that a dog to whom they had given a massive dose of morphine was capable of feeling pain. They said they thought it was not, for the dog's behavior seemed to suggest that its threshold response was reflexive, as the animal gave no indication that he was aware of what was happening during the test. I asked to see a demonstration. The dog they then showed me had been given an unusually large dose of morphine and he lolled in his restraining harness, drooling and paying not the slightest attention to commands, sudden noises, etc. Then they demonstrated that this animal made no visible response to shocks or ear pressure far above its normal pain threshold. But when I raised the setting of the electrical stimulator to a very high level and delivered a single strong stimulus to the dog's foreleg, he suddenly snapped at the electrode in a furious fashion. He immediately reverted to his previous inert posture and befuddled state, yet his quick response clearly indicated that the shock had produced an obnoxious sensation and that its source had been accurately localized.

Here is a second observation that still puzzles me and yet seems to support the opinion that pain perception must depend upon many other factors than stimulus intensity. During our studies of the analgesic properties of nitrous oxide, we used ourselves and a considerable number of medical students who volunteered to submit to the same tests. The subject to be tested first had a fine insulated wire with a bare tip temporarily soldered to an amalgam-filled tooth. The subject then lay on a padded table in a darkened room and a telegraph key was placed under his right hand. The wire was then connected with a stimulator in an adjoining room where someone could deliver single electrical pulses to the tooth, according to a definite schedule in which both the time intervals between pulses and the strength of each stimulation followed some prearranged sequence. The subject had no way of knowing when another stimulus would be given or what its intensity might be, but he was instructed to press the telegraph key once if he felt any sensation from the tooth and to press the telegraph key twice if the stab of pain in the tooth was about all he could tolerate. By matching his responses against the known intensity of each stimulus, it was easy to establish a curve for this subject, between his threshold and tolerance levels. When this chart had been completed, the subject was given nitrous oxide and oxygen for five minutes and then, while the gas administration continued, the same series of tests was repeated and a new threshold-to-tolerance curve was charted. In all subjects being tested for the first time the two charts clearly indicated that the gas inhalation had raised both the threshold and tolerance levels. This was exactly what we had expected to demonstrate. However, we found that if the same series of tests were repeated several times on the same subject the contrast between the two curves was much less evident. In other words, the subject's "nitrous oxide curve" tended to come closer and closer to his "normal curve," so that the threshold at which he perceived a stimulus was almost exactly the same, either with or without the nitrous oxide. His tolerance level under the gas influence usually tended to be somewhat higher than his "normal" level but definitely below the tolerance level shown by his original chart.

The only way we could account for this unexpected lowering of his threshold level was to assume that during the earlier tests he had learned exactly what to look for and so was better able to identify a threshold stimulus despite the mental confusion nitrous oxide always induces. We were not sure that this same explanation could account for the lowering of the tolerance level. My own subjective experience after repeated tests, however, was that the nitrous oxide gas definitely masked the obnoxious nature of the stimulus. But my previous experiences with strong stimuli had alerted me to some quality in the sensation, which I was able to interpret as a "threat" that any increase would cause more pain than I wished to tolerate.

The third observation involved a patient of Dr. Meares whom I considered the most reliable witness I had tested during my stay in Australia. This woman had been a physician before her marriage to a famous author. For many years she had suffered from back pain that had almost incapacitated her. She had been treated by many physicians and had spent long periods in hospitals under a variety of treatments including body casts, leg traction, and many forms of physiotherapy. None of these treatments or any form of back support had relieved her pain effectively. Some of her friends had suggested that she try treatments under hypnosis before she submitted to a surgical exploration for a "disc" or some other organic cause for the pain. She was reluctant to follow this advice because she had always associated hypnosis with quackery. Then it happened that her husband planned a trip to Italy to meet with his publishers and was anxious for her to accompany him. She wanted to go but was certain that the back pain would be intolerably aggravated during the trip whether she traveled by ship or by air. So, she decided to give hypnotic treatments a try, although she had no expectation that they could do her any good. To her surprise the treatments given her by Dr. Meares provided a great deal of pain relief and she learned from him how to self-induce a light hypnotic state after which her pain would be completely relieved for two hours or more and then would gradually return, although rarely to its former intensity. She was able to make the trip to Italy and had continued to use this form of "home treatment" ever since, supplemented from time to time by a trip to Melbourne for a treatment by Dr. Meares in which a deeper level of hypnosis seemed to afford more lasting relief. I asked this woman how often she used the self-induced hypnotic treatments and she said she rarely found it necessary to take the time to practice them. She thought that the fact that this therapeutic aid was always available to her helped make her residual back pain easier to bear. I was much impressed by this intelligent patient's story, and the way she described her method for inducing a light hypnotic state bolstered my hunch that muscular relaxation might be a factor in reducing her pain.

The fourth observation was made in New Delhi while I was visiting some neurophysiologists in the All-India Institute of Medical Sciences. They were trying to evaluate the claims that certain forms of yoga practice could exert some mysterious control over body functions. On this particular day we had a young yogi in the EEG room and were recording his brain waves while he was inducing a state of meditation, which he claimed would make him immune to pain. After he had been in the room a while the prevailing rhythms we were recording were of the alpha type and they did not desynchronize when we asked him questions or moved him about on the table. Then, we plunged one of his hands into a huge dishpan filled with ice cubes. The alpha rhythms were not altered during the forty-five minutes his hand remained in the ice water. This so-called "cold pressor test" is supposed to cause a normal person so much pain within two or three minutes after immersion that he is impelled to withdraw the hand from the ice water. Although I was impressed that this young yogi's alpha rhythm had not changed during the test, I did not think that his failure to remove his hand from the ice water was *proof* that he was feeling no pain. This opinion was challenged by some of the men present so I took a few minutes to relax and then put my hand in the pan for more than fourteen minutes, after which the experiment terminated. Naturally, the hand felt painfully cold but certainly not unbearably so.

I do not know enough about the various schools of yoga practice to discuss the claims of the few gurus I talked with in India, who told me that they could completely control pain by systematic exercises or meditation. But one thing that impressed me during my three visits to different ashrams that offered classes for students was the emphasis each teacher put on muscular relaxation. I had always thought of yoga exercises in terms of standing on one's head for a half hour or so at a time, or maintaining the lotus posture for long periods, but the classes I attended certainly did not encourage the student to remain in strained postures for any length of time, and each of these *asanas* was followed by a much longer *shavasana* in which complete muscular relaxation was encouraged. For example, after a brief *asana* the student was asked to lie back on a mat with hands at the side and all muscles relaxed. Then the student was instructed to take in a deep breath—hold it—and then let it slowly out again. After two long breaths the student rolled onto the right side and repeated the deep breathing, then onto the left side for the same two breaths, then again on the back for two more. Only then was another *asana* started. Thus, during a class period of an hour and a half there might be time for only six or seven *asanas*, with the rest of the time devoted to suggestions for muscular relaxation and the effects of breathing pure air during the *shavasana*.

Perhaps I am overemphasizing the resemblance between progressive muscular relaxation, hypnosis, and yoga exercises in their ability to modify pain perceptions. My point in calling attention to this possible resemblance is that I think all three claims are worthy of serious study by qualified neurophysiologists and such an investigation might well start with subjects trained in the art of progressive relaxation. It might be possible to establish correlations between brain waves, electromyograms, and tooth-pulp stimulation that would demonstrate some relationship between pain perception and degrees of muscular relaxation. If such correlations could be established, the same methods of investigation might be extended to subjects in hypnotic states of various degrees and the claims of yogis be put to a practical test.

17

The Pain Project

The final year of the Second World War was one of the most exciting and profitable periods of my life. I had the assistance of an efficient and enthusiastic staff who were teaching me the value of teamwork in the investigation of obscure clinical problems. Our wards were full of cases with every kind and degree of peripheral nerve injury. Our weekly conferences were spirited exchanges in which we were learning basic concepts in neurophysiology and psychology and better methods for doing nerve surgery, tendon transplants, and hand reconstructions. But the abrupt end of the war interrupted these activities as our group slowly began to disintegrate. Everybody, staff members and patients alike, wanted to get out of the service and go home. One by one the most valuable members of the staff left to return to civilian practice and, with their departure, much of the steam went out of our conferences. When I left military service a year later I was determined not to go back to private practice in Portland until I had made every effort to secure some research assignment that would enable me to assemble a similar team of experts willing to cooperate in an intensive study of human pain problems. The prospects did not seem bright and while I was looking around for a place to alight, I spent a few months as a guest professor in New York University Medical School and also accepted an invitation to give a few lectures in England during the summer of 1947.

Just before taking off for England I was offered the chair of surgery at the University of Oregon Medical School. I was surprised and pleased by this offer but I was afraid that the administrative duties in this assignment would divert me from my primary objective. However, the dean assured me that he wanted me to continue with my investigations and that I could delegate as much of the routine work of the department as I wished to a staff of my own selection. So, I accepted and happily took off for England. On my return to Portland at the end of the summer I was snowed under for a while with the task of assembling an efficient staff and getting departmental affairs organized. In the meantime, I let it be known among my faculty colleagues that I wanted to organize a "pain project" in which a team of investigators would conduct a simultaneous study of the physiological and psychological aspects of pain in our clinics and research laboratories. The response was enthusiastic and the team was soon organized by members drawn from

---

We therefore decided that we would take as our basic assumption the concept that nothing can properly be called pain unless it is consciously perceived as such.

---

both basic science and clinical departments. We agreed to meet once a week throughout the school year to build a common background of information relating to pain phenomena and to divide among ourselves the task of keeping abreast of the current literature pertinent to our shared interests. We would also supervise the work carried out by subgroups and individual members in the outpatient "Pain Clinic" and in the various research laboratories.

One of the first and most important tasks faced by this team was to decide just what we intended to investigate. We could not find a definition for "pain" that satisfied any of us but we all agreed, even the physiologists, that it was *not* a strictly physical "sensation" that could be defined by its anatomical and physiological substrates. What we wanted to study was the only kind of pain that human beings are concerned about and that is *the pain they consciously experience*. It seemed to us that there might be some justification for distinguishing between a "sensation" and its "perception" in the study of light and sound but that the attempt to make such a distinction in the case of pain was both artificial and misleading. We therefore decided that we would take as our basic assumption the concept that *nothing can properly be called pain unless it is consciously perceived as such.*

These seminar discussions were the mainspring of our investigation. In the next few chapters I will summarize some of the background information that influenced our interpretations. I will not attempt to report these discussions exactly as they occurred but rather as stories about individuals and their work. In putting so much emphasis on this background information it may seem that I underrate the importance of the individual studies being conducted simultaneously by members of our team (Appendix B).[1] All make important contributions to our understanding of pain phenomena. However, given that the central theme of this book is the evolving concept of pain, I will refer only to specific investigations that most directly bear on this theme. The only exception I will make to this plan of procedure is that I will begin with a description of our pain clinic and the difficulties we encountered in our efforts to study human pain problems.

Our pain clinic was set up in the outpatient department where once a week certain members of the team were to study selected cases suffering from "irritative nerve lesions." Before we opened this clinic we knew that we would be overwhelmed by cases clamoring for admission unless we started with a limited objective and accepted for study and treatment only those cases whose pain problem gave some promise of contributing to that objective. So, we decided to start by seeing what more we could learn about the usefulness of procaine in controlling chronic pain states when administered in any one of three ways: the injection of so-called "trigger points," the blocking of nerve pathways, and the intravenous injection of dilute solutions. By using these procedures we hoped to find clues as to why their beneficial effects so often persisted long after the procaine had been metabolized and eliminated. Finally, we intended to conduct experiments on cats to determine whether procaine had any central effect when it is administered intravenously in the same high dilution used for human cases.

---

[1]See Editor's Note in Appendix B.

Although these limited objectives have been pursued for years in the Pain Clinic, many questions about the effects of procaine on chronic pain states remain unanswered. We have learned to some extent which particular types of irritative nerve lesion are most likely to benefit from each form of procaine administration but we are still unable to predict in advance what its effects will be in a given case. We know that this drug is no panacea and yet it often confers a worthwhile degree of pain relief in cases that are resistant to any other form of treatment we know. Our observation of cases that have benefited from the injection of trigger points and nerve blocks has led us to think that the local action of procaine may reduce a pathological input to the nervous system that has contributed to the chronic pain state. For example, patients whose activities are severely limited by effort angina sometimes experience a material increase in their exercise tolerance after the sensitivity of trigger points in the muscles and fascia of their chest and shoulder has been reduced. Obviously, such injections are not directly affecting the cardiac lesion that presumably is causing the angina, so whatever degree of pain relief is conferred by the injections probably should be ascribed to a reduction of the sum total of the pathological input. This hypothesis has led us to search for, and to try to eliminate, any possible additive irritative foci in cases whose primary focus of irritation is inaccessible to direct treatment.

In the experimental laboratory we have been able to demonstrate that procaine has at least one central effect when administered intravenously in the same dilutions we use clinically. For example, the circulating drug actively depressed the responses to the stimulation of a known pain source (the tooth pulp) as they ascend in the reticular formation of the midbrain. The appearance of this depressant effect soon after the intravenous injection has been started may correlate with the remarkably prompt onset of subjective pain relief reported by patients being treated by an intravenous injection during a bout of pain. I can cite a case to illustrate this point after a brief description of the way we use this method of treatment.

In most clinics the dosage of procaine is estimated on the basis of this formula: "4 mg/kg body weight in a 0.2% solution administered by intravenous drip during a 20-minute period." We have not followed this formula exactly because the best results occur when the solution is given at a rate that elicits subjective reactions. When the drip rate is rapid, most patients report subjective sensations, a metallic taste in their mouths, a feeling of spreading warmth throughout the body and face, and a slight giddy sensation. If the prescribed rate of administration produces any of these systemic reactions the drip rate is not increased. However, if the patient fails to experience them, the drip rate is increased until it elicits sensations. We have used this form of treatment in a considerable number of patients without incident. We recognize the limitations of this method for the relief of pain, but it has served us well as an investigative tool and in emphasizing that procaine has a central as well as a peripheral action.

Mr. C. first reported to the pain clinic in 1948. His chief complaints were "lightning pains" in his legs associated with uncontrollable jerking of the legs during the attacks of pain. He had been diagnosed with tabes dorsalis at least twelve years previously, but the treatment he had been given in the syphilis clinic had not altered his "tabetic crises." At the time we first saw this man his shocks of pain were almost continuous and he had been referred to the Pain Clinic for a series of procaine injections. We had no real expectations of being able to relieve his suffering but he was so desperately anxious to try the injections that we accepted him for treatment. For the first few weeks we could observe no change in his condition, although he thought that perhaps his pains were a little less severe. Then he began to have two or three days after each injection during which he was completely free from both the pain and the jerking of his limbs. Finally, a point was reached at which he remained free from pain from one treatment to the next. Over the years there were times when he did not have to return for another injection for three to six weeks. The main objection to this regimen of intermittent treatments was that the Pain Clinic convened only on Tuesdays and if his pain came back four or five days before he could get an intravenous injection it seemed that the cumulative benefit of the previous treatments was lost and it might require a month or two of weekly treatments before the period of pain relief would again extend over a two-week interval.

I have observed Mr. C. on several occasions when he was having pain attacks. With every shock of pain he would wince and his legs would jerk violently. There was no question in the mind of anyone observing him at such times that his pain was extremely severe. When the intravenous drip was started the drug effect was apparent within a very few seconds. Simultaneous with his statement that he "felt" the drug effects, he reported that his pain had gradually faded. We observed a rapid quieting of the leg jerking and a change in his facial expression as his anxious look was replaced by a pleased look of satisfaction. The remarkable feature of this drug effect was that it occurred before he could have absorbed more than a small fraction of the total dosage. However, none of the physicians in the pain clinic felt that these changes were purely "psychic" in origin or that this man showed any of the signs of a physiological dependency on the procaine, such as the opiate addict shows for his drug.

On one occasion the clinic nurse forgot to put the ampoule of 2% procaine into each of the bottles of normal salt solution used in the treatments given on that particular day. Mr. C. was one of the patients who received only normal saline in his intravenous drip. He reported back the following week to say that he had had a "terrible" seven days of suffering, with his pains and leg jerkings as severe as they had ever been. He said he was sure that there must have been something the matter with the solution he had been given the week previously because it had not done him the slightest bit of good. Of course, it is apparent that the procaine injections had not "cured" this man's tabetic crises, yet a treatment every two weeks or so was all that it took to make his life bearable.

Everyone who has worked in the pain clinic has learned much about human pain problems, their various types, their urgency, and their destructive potentials. And it may be that they have also learned an important therapeutic principle that is particularly applicable to chronic pain states in which the source is unknown or inaccessible to direct attack: Don't ever give up attempts to lessen a patient's burden of pain. If the source is not removable, keep whittling down all possible additive factors and the pain may be reduced in intensity.

18

The Philosophers and Johannes Müller

As the members of our team searched for a satisfactory definition for pain we were amazed by the number and variety of definitions to be found in dictionaries and scientific textbooks. According to one definition pain was an "affective" state of the mind; according to another, it was a special body sense. One definition emphasized the "protective" aspect of pain; another stressed only its "destructive" potentialities. A dictionary might say that pain is "uneasiness of mind" and equate it with grief and anxiety, while a physiologist defined pain as "the psychical adjunct of an imperative protective reflex." As we examined three various definitions it seemed to us that there was some truth in all of them. Nevertheless, we had the impression that each authority was defining only that aspect of pain that he could see most clearly from the particular point of view conditioned by his early training and professional interests. The situation reminded us of the old tale of the three blind men, each of whom described an elephant in terms of the single part of the body he had palpated. Each of the three descriptions had truth in it, yet they all failed to depict a dynamic whole. The same fault seemed to us to apply to the available definitions for pain. But if we sought a more satisfactory definition we ought to know something about the original meaning of the word and the historical background for its subsequent interpretations.

The word pain is derived from the Greek *poine* and the Latin *poena*, both of which signified "a penalty or punishment." In common with most primitive peoples, the early Greeks believed that their pantheon of gods controlled the behavior of each human being by dispensing rewards and punishments according to the person's merits or to their own whims. The highest rewards the gods could confer on one of their favorites were the physical perfections and personal attainments that afforded the person the greatest *pleasure*. The cruelest punishments they could inflict were the deprivations and physical afflictions that gave the most *pain*. Thus, "reward and punishment" and "pleasure and pain" came to be linked together among the "great ideas" with which every philosopher must contend in any consideration of human behavior. Apparently, none of the famous Greek philosophers classified pain among the special senses of the body. Instead, they maintained that pain was the antithesis of pleasure and they spoke of both as being "qualities of the soul."[1]

None of the members of our team felt qualified to say what the philosophers meant by the word "soul." It is evidently not synonymous with such words as "spirit" or "mind" as we use them today. Furthermore, the philosophers apparently endowed human beings with more than one kind of soul, types that might be termed mortal, immortal, and universal. In our effort to understand the meaning of this word we read some of the works of the Greek philosophers and found in them many concepts that might have a bearing on our interpretation of pain. In *Timaeus*, Plato wrote:

> God took such of the primary triangles which were smooth and straight and adapted by their perfection to produce fire and water, air and earth; these I say, he separated from their kinds and mingling them in due proportions, one with another, made "marrow" out of them to be the universal seed for the whole race of mankind, and in this seed he planted and enclosed the souls, and in the original distribution gave to the marrow as many and varied forms as the different kinds of souls were hereafter to receive. That which, like a field, was to receive the divine seed he made round in every way and called that portion of the marrow "brain" intending that, when an animal was perfected the vessel containing this substance should be the head but that which was to contain the remaining and mortal part of the soul should be distributed into figures at once round and elongated, and he called them by the name "marrow"; and to these, as to anchors, fastening the bonds of the soul, he proceeded to fashion around them the entire framework of our body, constructing for the marrow, first of all, a complete covering of bone.

---

[1]*Editor's Note:* For a brief annotated introduction to the ideas on pain discussed by the Greek philosophers, I recommend that the reader consult "The Greek debate on the heart, brain and pain," Chapter 2 in Keele KD, *Anatomies of Pain.* Oxford: Blackwell, 1957, pages 16–40.

Plato speculated freely about the mysteries of birth, growth, aging, and death as parts of the "process of becoming." He said that the triangles in the bodies of young animals were "new and sharp as the newly laid keel of a vessel just off the stocks," so that when the young animal ingested food, his triangles could easily cut up and fashion into their own kind, the older and weaker triangles constituting the ingested food. Of this process, he wrote:

> And in this way the animal grows great, being nourished by a multitude of similar particles. . . . But, when the roots of the triangles are loosened, by having undergone many conflicts with many things in the course of time, they are no longer able to cut and assimilate the food which enters but are themselves easily divided by the bodies that come in from without. In this way the animal is overcome and decays, and this affection is called old age. And, at last, when the bonds by which the triangles are united, no longer hold, and are parted by the strain of existence, they in turn loosen the bonds of the soul and she, obtaining a natural release, flies away with joy. *For that which takes place according to nature is pleasant, but that which is contrary to nature is painful.*

Aristotle also spoke of pain and pleasure as being "passions of the soul," and he failed to list either one among the special senses that he said distinguished animals from vegetative forms of life. Yet, he evidently felt that the relationship was close because he wrote: "Wherever there is sensation there is also pain or pleasure and where these two feelings are there is necessarily desire." He believed that there were only five special senses—touch, taste, smell, sight, and hearing. Of these, the sense of touch was the "primary" one because even the most primitive forms of animal life lacking in other special senses could respond to contact stimuli. He said of touch: "The loss of this one sense alone must bring about the death of an animal." He believed that touch and taste represented a lower order than the other three special senses and his reason for rating them lower was that an animal having no other senses must come into direct contact with the external object before it could be identified. Smell, sight, and hearing were of a higher order because they permitted recognition of the external object from a distance. As to the nature of sensation he wrote: "By a 'sense' is meant what has the power of receiving into itself the sensible form of things without matter." To clarify his meaning he mentioned the imprint that a signet ring can make in soft wax. Although the imprint lacks the iron and gold of the ring itself, it so faithfully reproduces its "sensible form"

As to the first question, Müller was inclined to doubt that every type of sensation that can be elicited by skin stimulation had its own specialized sensory receptor. His seventh law raises the second question. He wrote: "It is not known whether the essential cause of the peculiar energy of each nerve of sense is situated in the nerve itself, or in the parts of the brain and spinal cord with which it is connected; but it is certain that the central portions of the nerves included in the encephalon are susceptible of their peculiar sensations, independently of the more peripheral portion of the nervous cords which form the means of communication with the external organs of sense." In support of this view he mentions phantom limb pains and other definite sensations that amputees often ascribe to distant parts of an absent limb. Müller attempted to answer the third question in his ninth and tenth laws. In the ninth he said that the projection of sensation to particular parts of the body and its subjective qualities are ascribable to associated ideas the person has learned from past experience. Finally, in the tenth law he said: "The mind not only perceives the sensations and interprets them according of the ideas previously obtained, but it has a direct influence upon them, imparting to them intensity."

Müller is credited with having enunciated the "law of specific nerve energies." It is usually interpreted as meaning that each kind of sensation is due to the activation of a specifically adapted sensory neuron. Müller's own words make it clear that he questioned this interpretation, but his penetrating commentaries seem to have been overlooked both then and now. At least, the immediate effect of Müller's teachings was to start scientists on an intensive search for the "specific" sensory neuron subserving each of the many sensations that can be elicited by skin stimulation. This search was aided by the development of new techniques for cutting and staining tissue sections and by the development of microscope lenses with higher resolving power. It could then be seen that human skin is supplied by sensory fibers of many different sizes, whose terminal arborizations ended in a variety of morphologically distinct types of terminal. The endings of each sensory fiber were characteristic for that particular fiber in being as like each other as the flowers on a single stalk. These endings ranged in complexity from tiny, undifferentiated, "naked" terminals in intimate contact with tissue cells, to complex and highly organized receptor "organs." In addition, it was noted that each type of receptor organ might vary in size and complexity, so that for a time it seemed that there were plenty of these distinct types of ending to account for every kind of sensation that can be elicited by skin stimulation. Yet, the task of identifying the particular ending that subserved one particular sensation was complicated because sensory fibers of different size intermingled freely in their terminal arborizations and several types of ending were found in close proximity in areas of microscopic size.

The technical difficulties involved in proving that each type of sensation depended on the activation of a particular receptor neuron were soon apparent. The search for the specific sensory unit subserving "pleasure" was the first to be abandoned, then the unit for "itch," until finally, many physiologists were inclined to give up the whole task as hopelessly difficult. Then, in 1885, Blix and Goldscheider, working independently, announced their discovery that skin sensibility is not everywhere uniform but has a "punctate" distribution (Blix 1885; Goldscheider 1885). In testing their own skin, each man had found tiny spots from which mechanical stimulation elicited a remarkably vivid sensation of "cold." Mechanical pressure on other spots gave rise to a vague sensation of "warmth." In between these "heat" and "cold" spots were many more from which a sensation of "pain" could be elicited by relatively light pressure, while from all intervening areas the same stimulus produced a sensation of "touch." No sensation other than these four types could be demonstrated by this form of testing, and the natural assumption was that there were only four "pure" sensations to be derived from skin stimulation and that beneath each "skin spot" would be found the specifically adapted sensory receptor for one sensation only.

This assumption became the basis for what was called the "punctate theory." Its main postulate was that cold, heat, touch, and pain must represent "primary" sensations, each subserved by a single specialized sensory unit. From these "four modalities of cutaneous sensibility" all other sensations derived from skin stimulation were supposed to be compounded. In 1895 von Frey published a long series of experimental observations in support of the punctate theory (von Frey 1894, 1895). He used hairs and bristles of graded stiffness to demonstrate that the amount of pressure necessary to elicit the appropriate sensation from each skin spot was approximately the same in every test. He interpreted this finding as indicating that the four kinds of receptor ending had their own characteristic thresholds and, presumably, other equally unique physiological properties. Von Frey maintained that any reasonably intelligent person should be able to distinguish between "true pain" and mere "unpleasantness." He emphasized this distinction because he was convinced that pain was a primary sensation, while unpleasantness, like pleasure, was merely an "affective state of mind."

As the punctate theory gained favor, each of the four modalities of cutaneous sensibility was assigned its own specific receptor. Pain was ascribed to the activation of small, nonmyelinated sensory fibers with naked terminals; cold was ascribed to Krause's end-bulbs; heat to the organ of Ruffini; and touch to Meissner corpuscles, Merkel's disks, and the basket-endings around hair follicles. These assignments were difficult to substantiate experimentally and there was considerable disagreement among investigators as to which particular types of ending subserved sensations of heat, cold, and touch. But almost all the researchers agreed that the naked terminals of the smallest of the sensory fibers (later called "C" fibers) were specific for pain sensation. One of the most persuasive of the arguments in favor of this view was that the pulp of the teeth, the tympanic membrane of the ear, and the central part of the cornea of the eye, all known to be exquisitely sensitive to pain and said to be lacking in touch and temperature sensibility, were exclusively supplied by fine sensory fibers with naked terminals.

Although Goldscheider is usually remembered as one of the founders of the punctate theory, it is of considerable interest that his subsequent studies led him to doubt that the so-called "pain fibers" either were the sole source for pain sensation or exclusively subserved this single sensation. For example, he found that extremely light contact to the central part of the cornea of his own eye elicited a distinct sensation of touch that was devoid of any painful quality. He also observed that when pressing on a "touch spot," a slight increase in the pressure caused the sensation to change from touch to pain. The transition was so gradual that he doubted that any specific fiber for pain had suddenly been activated when its threshold had been reached. As late as 1936, Woollard, an authority on the microscopic anatomy of the skin, attempted to dispose of Goldscheider's argument in these words: "It is a common enough observation, mentioned by others, to find a thin fiber entering into a nerve ending. This additional 'accessory' ending had, on the ground of its thin non-medullated character, been regarded as sympathetic (Woollard 1936). It may, however, and in our judgement, even more probably, be regarded as an accessory nerve of pain. It is not suggested that a receptor changed its sensation. In the eye this function is supplied by the fifth nerve, which furnishes pain receptors and pain only, to the eye, itself. In the case of the internal ear the same function is undertaken by the seventh nerve. The secondary fiber exercises the same function for hairs, Meissner corpuscles, Pacinian corpuscles and other deep endings."

The concept of pain as a "primary" sensation subserved by a specifically adapted "pain fiber" has been difficult to displace. Among the first steps in this process has been the demonstration of touch and temperature sensibility in the cornea; another has been the discovery that the activation of sensory fibers much larger than C fibers causes pain sensations. A third step has been provided by evidence that there are routes in the spinal cord, other than the "pain and temperature tract," by which incoming sensory patterns can reach perceptual levels to be interpreted as pain. And there are more steps to come.

19

The "Reticular Formation"

During the first few years of our pain project, the members of the team gradually became aware that a revolution was occurring in neurophysiology. The first thing we noticed was that it was becoming increasingly difficult to review all the current literature in this field. Although we divided this task among us, and the seminar discussions could assist us all in digesting the new information, we were overwhelmed by an avalanche of new discoveries and interpretations. What made it all so difficult was that we were finding it necessary to reorganize most of the concepts we had always thought were founded on scientifically established facts and basic to an understanding of neurophysiology. Work on the reticular formation helped us immensely in this reorganization.

The primary concern of classical neurology was to identify the structures in the nervous system constituting the great inflow and outflow systems that maintain the body in harmony with its internal and external environments. Attention focused first on the peripheral nerves and the long-fiber tracts within the spinal cord and brain that connected the massive collections of nerve cells constituting the neuron pools concerned with sensory input and motor output. The fiber tracts connecting these neuron pools resembled the peripheral nerves in that they were composed of compact bundles of insulated nerve fibers. Their structure indicated they were capable of rapidly transmitting "messages" from one neuron pool to the next with no loss of their specific content. In fact, these tracts looked so much like great cables of insulated telephone wires that the "telephone exchange" was chosen as

155

the model for the central nervous system and the way it was supposed to operate. In turn, the use of this model fostered the notion that both sensory and motor messages were transmitted from one neuron to the next, extending in a single chain from source to destination. The diagram of the "simple reflex arc" implied that the relationship between a stimulus and its response (SR) was always direct and immediate, while the diagram of the "three-neuron pain pathway" was an affirmation of faith in sensory "specificity."

The early investigators were aware that the central nervous system contained billions of nerve cells outside the sensory and motor systems, but the available techniques were not well adapted for elucidating their functions. For example, there were many small nerve cells with short, interlacing branches alongside the fiber tracts in the spinal cord and huge clusters of them throughout the length of the brainstem. A particularly large mass formed a dense reticulum around the aqueduct of Sylvius in the midbrain, which forms the upper end of the brainstem. In fact, this mass of cells in the core of the midbrain was so large that the sensory and motor fiber tracts had to detour around them. This diffuse collection of nerve cells in the spinal cord and brainstem was named the "reticular formation" (RF). There was nothing about the arrangement of their branches to suggest that they served as part of any conducting system, and in the anesthetized brains used in most of the early investigations they showed little or no electrical activity. Some research workers thought that the RF served principally as a supporting reticulum, or "filler," packed around the main fiber tracts and nuclear masses as excelsior is sometimes used to pack around dishes in a barrel. (I have even heard the midbrain RF jocularly referred to as the "manure pile" of the brain.) However, one thing was known about a particular part of the RF that should have warned investigators not to dismiss the functions of the RF so lightly: injuries to the RF at the level of the medulla oblongata were almost always immediately fatal, with the animal dying from cardiac or respiratory failure.

In 1932 William F. Allen read a paper before the Washington Academy of Science entitled "Formatio Reticularis and Reticulospinal Tracts." His report was based on a five-year study of the functions of the RF and it began in these words: "It is known from embryology that most of the leftover cells of the brain stem and spinal cord which are not concerned in the formation of motor root nuclei and purely sensory relay nuclei are utilized in the production of the formatio reticularis. This is a very old structure phylogenetically. It is but little differentiated in the lower vertebrates, where it apparently serves as an effective mechanism which enables these animals to adapt themselves properly to their various inside and outside conditions. In the higher vertebrates there is but little reticular formation in the spinal cord, but considerable in both the median and lateral portions of the medulla, pons and midbrain, where for the most part it exists anatomically in its original undifferentiated state" (Allen 1932). He mentioned the functions of the portion in the medulla in controlling cardiac and respiratory functions and then listed the many other functions performed by the RF as suggested by his studies. He believed that the RF received an input from all levels of the nervous system and that its output was equally widespread in its regulating influence on endocrine balance, the posture and movement of muscles, and all the many body activities serving to maintain the body in harmony with its internal and external environment. Allen's contribution was of major importance but its significance seems to have been overlooked for more than a decade until Magoun and his co-workers began to use unanesthetized preparations in their effort to elaborate the functions of what they originally called "Allen's Alley."

Morruzzi and Magoun (1949) had been trying to determine the role of the "reticular formation" (RF) in regulating the motor outflow of the extrapyramidal system. In the anesthetized animal brain, the RF is relatively "silent" electrically but in unanesthetized preparations they found the RF to be extraordinarily active and to be transmitting a massive sensory input to higher levels in the brain. Their evidence indicated that collateral branches from fibers in the classical sensory tracts entered the RF throughout the length of the brainstem and this sensory input was then carried upward over multisynaptic chains to reach many distant parts of the brain. This meant that the sensory input from all parts of the body was reaching the brain by two quite separate routes. The portion carried by the classical route to the relay nuclei of the thalamus was delivered solely to the "specific" sensory areas of the cerebral cortex, while the portion ascending by the RF route was apparently reaching the brain as a whole.

To find out how these separate sensory inputs might affect brain functioning, Morruzzi and Magoun performed two critical experiments.

First, they blocked the RF route by making a massive lesion in the core of the midbrain. This lesion destroyed most of the RF cells but not the classical sensory tracts. Animals subjected to this procedure remained in a persistent state of deep coma as long as they could be kept alive by tube feeding. Not only were they behaviorally "unconscious," but their brain waves showed the long slow changes in electrical potential that are characteristic of "sleep." Although they demonstrated that responses to stimulation were reaching the specific cortices over the classical route, no form of stimulation, no matter how intense, could arouse the animal from its state of coma. In the second experiment, the classical sensory tracts were divided just caudal to the thalamus, thus leaving their collaterals to the RF intact. Animals subjected to this procedure were not rendered comatose but seemed to alternate between sleep and wakefulness in an apparently normal fashion. When they were asleep and their EEG recordings showed the typical "sleep waves" a sudden noise, a bright light or a pinch awakened them and the sleep waves were promptly replaced by the desynchronized pattern of activity that characterizes the "alert" state of the brain.

This experimental evidence indicated that the sensory pathway ascending in the RF had more to do with "arousal" of the animal and the maintenance of consciousness than did the classical sensory route. Morruzzi and Magoun named this newly discovered sensory pathway, the "reticular activating system" (RAS). They said of it: "The presence of a steady background of less intense activity within this cephalically directed brainstem system, contributed either by liminal inflows from peripheral receptors or preserved intrinsically, may be an important factor contributing to the maintenance of the waking state, and that absence of such activity in it may predispose to sleep." In this same report the authors suggested that the sleep-inducing influence of barbiturate drugs might be due to a blocking of sensory conduction in the multisynaptic RAS pathway rather than, as had been previously assumed, to a depression of function in the cortical cells in the specific sensory areas of the brain. This discovery delighted me because it seemed to put in perspective the concept of pain based on a "three-neuron pain pathway" to the sensory cortex and to vindicate our decision that "nothing can properly be called pain unless it is consciously recognized as such."

In 1935 Bremer noted that when an animal's brain was isolated from the rest of the nervous system by a transection of the brainstem in the upper portion of the midbrain, the brain waves promptly changed from the low-voltage desynchronized type characteristic of the alert brain to the long, slow sleep waves (Bremer 1935). He attributed this altered state of the brain to the fact that it was not receiving any sensory input to keep it awake. He confirmed this impression by making transections at lower levels to permit sensory input from the trigeminal nerves to reach the brain and found that under these conditions the brain waves were not altered. However, the additional severance of the trigeminal nerves promptly changed the brain waves to the sleep type. Based on these observations, Bremer concluded that the maintenance of consciousness was incompatible with an absence of any sensory input to the brain. This discovery had implications beyond those relating to the mechanisms underlying states of sleep and consciousness. Neurophysiologists were suddenly made aware of the importance of research on the unanesthetized brain for understanding how it might function as a "mind." They already possessed precision techniques for inserting tiny wire electrodes into any part of the animal brain, even in single nerve cells, and could use them to stimulate a particular locus or make graphic records of the electrical changes occurring from moment to moment. If these techniques could be adapted for use in unanesthetized brains, perhaps they could determine what was happening in the brain of a normal, unrestrained animal as it performed its various functions or responded to test conditions. Its behavior under these different situations would provide clues as to its motivations; if at the same time a graphic record could be made of the simultaneous changes in brain activity, it might eventually be possible to establish correlations between brain activity and psychological processes. What an exciting prospect! Here was a method of investigation that offered promise of illuminating such important psychological processes as consciousness, attention, emotions, learning, and purpose.

The pursuit of this goal is already under way. The techniques for making permanent implants of fine wire electrodes in the animal brain are well established. All that needs to be said here is that their presence apparently does little damage to the brain tissue nor does it seem to alter the animal's normal behavior once it has recovered from the minor operation required for the electrode placements. The multiple wires leading to the sites selected for study lead to a plastic button fastened securely to the skull and containing a multiple-lead jack into which can be plugged, at will, a long, flexible cable of wires leading to an oscilloscope. The permanent presence of the plastic button seems to cause the animal no discomfort or inconvenience. This can be said with reasonable assurance because exactly this same procedure has been employed for human patients suffering from epilepsy or other brain disorders and they say that the presence of the plastic button is neither unpleasant nor inconvenient. In the case of certain animals, such as the monkey, ingenious methods have been employed to avoid even the minor restraints imposed by the wire cable. In such instances, the implanted electrodes lead through the plastic button to a small pack on the animal's back and they can be activated by remote control. José Delgado has used this technique on a colony of monkeys at Yale (Delgado 1954). In a large cage, behind one-way glass, these monkeys go about their normal activities without being aware that they are under observation. Then, by remote control, it is possible to stimulate any part of the brain of a particular monkey. Depending on the placement of the electrode, it is possible to waken a sleeping animal or promptly put an alert one to sleep, tame a vicious animal that is attacking another, or cause a placid individual to viciously attack a cage mate. By selecting particular areas for stimulation, the researcher may cause the animal to salivate, defecate, have a penile erection, suddenly arrest its activity, or exhibit all the evidences of "shock." These uncanny manipulations of the experimental animal not only involve the body functions but seem to change the emotions as well.

Drugs have been used as an alternative to electrical stimulation. An ingenious assembly called a "chemitrode" allows a minute quantity of some drug to be injected into a particular area of the animal's brain. Instead of a stimulating electrode, an extremely small tube extends from the site for injection to a tiny pump enclosed in a capsule attached to the animal's back. This pump can be activated by remote control to deposit some of the drug solution at the chosen site and its effect on the animal behavior can be observed or recorded on movie film without distracting the animal's attention. In one of Delgado's experiments a chemitrode was introduced into the brain of "Ali," the boss bully of a colony of monkeys. At the site selected for injection, a minute amount of the solution had the power to stop Ali as he was making a savage attack on an offending cage mate and alter his emotional behavior from rage to placid equanimity. A lever was installed within the cage that, when pulled, activated the pump and deposited enough drug in Ali's brain to change his behavior. It did not take the other monkeys long to discover how to use this lever to change Ali from a bullying boss to a docile companion.

The evidence that the stimulation of localized areas of the brain may alter emotions as well as behavior has not been entirely limited to experiments on animals. Implant electrodes have been used for both diagnosis and treatment of human patients suffering from obscure types of epilepsy and other brain disorders. Naturally, the selection of patients for this form of brain stimulation must be made with extreme care, and the use of multiple implants can be justified only in the search for the exact site of an epileptic focus or in the attempt to find a spot where stimulation may relieve the pain of a patient suffering from an inoperable cancer.

Yet, enough patients in many different psychiatric clinics have been tested by direct brain stimulation techniques to permit the conclusion that the behavioral manifestations of such emotional states as fear, anger, malaise, pleasure, and pain are associated with subjective feelings meriting these designations. In certain instances remote control stimulation of the brain of a patient in the midst of a violent psychotic seizure characterized by rage and aggressive behavior has quickly produced a state of mild euphoria. In the Psychiatric Clinic at Tulane, Robert Heath has equipped a few psychotic patients with portable self-stimulators (Heath and Mickle 1960). Usually, such a patient wears a device with three buttons that is attached to a belt. When the patient feels an "attack" coming on, he can repeatedly press the particular button that affords the most relief of symptoms and that might prevent the seizure from developing further.

All these observations are of enormous interest to all students of "mind-brain" relationships, but the ones I have described so far are only the most spectacular and by no means the most important ones. In research laboratories all over the world there are now assembled splendidly equipped research teams that include neurophysiologists, psychologists, pharmacologists, and clinicians who are pooling their skills and insights in experiments on a great variety of laboratory animals with the hope of establishing reliable correlations between patterns of brain activity and such psychological processes as attention, memory, and learning. To this team effort the neurophysiologists and anatomists contribute their skills in the exact placement of stimulating and recording electrodes; the psychologists add their sophisticated methods for analyzing behavior and all types of conditioning; the pharmacologists contribute their knowledge of such drugs as reserpine, LSD, and chlorpromazine, which can modify behavior. A prodigious amount of information has been derived from the use of these combined techniques, but even when all the available knowledge has been pooled it is apparent that the goal of correlating brain activities with mental processes is still far off. What is becoming clear, however, is that no functioning of the alert brain is any simple "from-here-to-there affair" but a "transaction" of enormous complexity moving forward in an established time sequence and, apparently, according to a definite teleological design.

20

Two Blind Alleys: Nerve Irritation and "Zombies"

W hen the pain project was first organized we hoped to devise laboratory experiments that might give us more information about the neural substrates for pain and the nature of nerve "irritation," but we had no clear ideas as to how to begin either line of investigation. Our decision that "nothing can properly be called pain unless it is consciously perceived as such" seemed to raise insuperable obstacles to the first line of investigation because we did not know how we could be sure that a particular pattern of sensory impulses (the "signal") gave rise to a "pain perception." Nor did any of us know what the nature of nerve "irritation" might be or how to create a "focus of chronic irritation." The effort to get around these obstacles greatly broadened the scope of our seminar discussions and led us into a few blind alleys in the laboratory as well as into more productive lines of investigation. Among our early ventures were two that were highly instructive and yet had to be dropped for want of definite leads to more conclusive findings. I wish to give a brief description of these ventures because both had points of interest bearing on our interpretive problems.

Nerve Irritation

My search for a nerve irritant that might give rise to the causalgic type of pain began many years ago. In 1938 Tönnies had demonstrated what were called "posterior root reflexes" in sensory nerves (Tönnies 1938). When he applied a single shock to a sensory nerve he could record a response coming back down the nerve that had apparently originated in neuron pools within the spinal cord. A year later Barron and Matthews (1938) had shown that these dorsal root reflexes were exaggerated under certain abnormal conditions such as cooling the animal. They also suggested that these reflexes might have something to do with creating causalgic states in humans. In 1941 Dow and Anderson joined me in an effort to test this suggestion. We were able to create an indolent and apparently painful ulcer on a dog's foreleg by injecting a drop or two of croton oil into the sheath of its superficial radial nerve. After fifteen to forty days we compared the dorsal root reflexes of such an animal with those of normal dogs, making our tests at both normal body temperatures and after cooling. Of course, we could not be sure that a chronic leg ulcer induces "causalgia" in a dog, but in any event, we were unable to demonstrate that the presence of an ulcer could alter the dorsal root reflexes.

Some earlier observations reported by Dusser de Barenne encouraged me to continue the search for a nerve irritant. When he applied strychnine to the spinal cord of a cat, near where the posterior root enters, the cat behaved as if the cutaneous area supplied by this root had become hypersensitive (Dusser de Barenne 1931). The influence of the strychnine on cutaneous sensibility was relatively transient, but this observation suggested that if one could find some substance that would irritate sensory neurons for a longer period, a persistent state of hyperesthesia might develop, similar to that seen in the causalgic state. One substance that offered some promise of supplying the sustained irritation I was seeking was the aluminum cream that Dr. Kopeloff and his wife were using on the motor cortex of monkeys to induce epileptiform seizures (Kopeloff 1955).

The Kopeloffs had found that when they applied a little of this substance to a limited area of a monkey's motor cortex, the animal subsequently began to have convulsive seizures resembling those exhibited by humans suffering from the Jacksonian type of epilepsy. The sequence of events that developed after the application followed this sequence. For many days or weeks there was no observable change in the monkey's behavior. Then it began to have occasional jerkings and twitchings of the muscles in one part of its body. If the aluminum cream had been deposited over the "leg area" of the motor cortex, the muscular contractions first appeared in the leg of the opposite side; if the cream had been localized over the "hand area," the motor changes began in the hand. As time went on, the motor seizures spread to involve the ipsilateral limb, then extended to the contralateral limbs, and finally the whole body musculature became involved in recurrent, generalized convulsions. Thereafter, each attack exhibited that regular "march" of events that is so characteristic of Jacksonian epilepsy. Kopeloff found that if he removed the aluminum cream and excised the cortex directly beneath its area of application, he could prevent the development of the epileptiform attacks, provided this procedure was done within the first day or two after the material had been applied. However, if the irritant was left on the cortex for three or more days, not even the most extensive cortical excisions could prevent the subsequent development of the seizures. The implications drawn from these observations were as follows: For a day or two the irritation caused by the aluminum cream had affected only the cortical cells in its immediate vicinity, but then the "irritation" had spread to involve nerve cells much deeper in the substance of the brain. Once this had happened there seemed to be no way to prevent an inexorable "buildup" and "spread" of the irritation until it had finally manifested its presence in explosive attacks of muscular contractions, first exhibited locally and then generally.

Almost exactly the same sequence of events had been described earlier by the Russian scientist Speranskii after he had frozen a small area of a dog's motor cortex with carbon dioxide snow (Speranskii 1936). He had bored a hole in the dog's skull and had frozen the underlying cortex without opening the dura. If he removed the small block of damaged cortical cells within one or two days after the freezing, no subsequent trouble developed, but if he delayed the excision any longer the dog subsequently began to have Jacksonian epileptic attacks and eventually died in status epilepticus. I had read the English translation of Speranskii's book, which described this experiment as the starting point for an amazing series of experiments on the brains and spinal cords of animals upon which Speranskii based a theory of medicine in which he attributed all kinds of disease syndromes to nerve "irritation." I felt that the all-inclusiveness of his interpretations was prejudicial to the acceptance of his observations at their face value. So, I was glad to see that the Kopeloff experiments had at least confirmed his observations.

My observations of industrial accident cases had indicated that Jacksonian epilepsy may develop in humans after almost any kind of cortical injury. Any operation on the brain that requires opening the dura, even the most carefully performed, seems to carry some risk of the subsequent development of this type of epilepsy. Although extensive scars involving the motor area are more likely to cause epileptic attacks than are small ones, no one can predict in advance whether a particular lesion will serve as a chronic source of irritation. In this respect cortical lesions resemble peripheral nerve lesions in that neither gross nor microscopic examinations of the scar can distinguish the occasional one that will cause future trouble from the many others that do not. The two types of lesion are also alike in other features. They both have the capacity to disorganize function in distant neural circuits within the central nervous system and in both types the removal of the original scar may fail to stop the central perturbation of function.

It struck me that if the aluminum cream the Kopeloffs were using possessed the irritative potential of the very worst of cortical lesions, perhaps it might be used to create a state simulating "causalgia" if it was applied to peripheral nerves or posterior root ganglia. Early in 1947, while I was a guest professor in the Anatomy Department of the New York University Medical School, Dr. Margaret Kennard was working in the same laboratories. I knew that she had done some of the surgery on the Kopeloff monkeys and I asked her where I might see a monkey that had developed Jacksonian attacks due to the application of the aluminum cream. She took me to the animal quarters and showed me a monkey she had operated on about six weeks previously and which was just beginning to have Jacksonian attacks. I watched this animal for some time but could observe nothing abnormal about its behavior. I remarked that I wished I could see it during one of its attacks. Dr. Kennard answered, "You want to see him in an attack? I hate to pick on the little fellow but perhaps I can show you one." With a long stick poked through the cage bars she teased the monkey until it became greatly excited, chattering and jumping about in the cage. When she stopped teasing him, the monkey sat quietly on the floor of the cage and it seemed that nothing was going to happen. Suddenly, his right arm and hand began to twitch and Dr. Kennard exclaimed, "Here it comes." The arm jerking became more violent, the head turned sharply to the right and the right leg started jerking. Then the head swung left and the left arm and leg began jerking. Within a few seconds the entire body was involved in violent clonic muscular contractions that persisted for several more seconds. When the attack was over the monkey remained quiet, as if dazed, and then it resumed its normal activities.

The following year Dr. Kennard joined our research team at the University of Oregon Medical School and she brought with her some of the aluminum cream that had been prepared by Dr. Lenore Kopeloff. We intended to use some of this material on the peripheral nerves, posterior roots, or the spinal cords of cats to see what effect it might have on these animals. During applications to the monkey brain the cream was covered with a plastic disk to prevent its diffusion over wider areas. However, this method for limiting the site of application could not be used on the nerves or cord of the cat because of their small size. Instead, Dr. Kennard used a tuberculin syringe and needle to gradually inject 0.1 cc or less of the solution near the posterior aspect of the lumbar enlargement of the spinal cord. Although the dosage was small and could be expected to affect the posterior quadrants of the cord more than the anterior quadrants or the posterior root fibers, there was nothing to prevent the spread of the material in any direction within the limits of the dural space. For a few days after such an injection, the cat showed no alteration of its normal behavior. Then the animal began to develop a hypersensitiveness of the skin over both hind legs. This cutaneous hyperesthesia gradually spread until it involved both hind legs and tail and seemed to extend a segment or so higher than the level of injection. Blowing on the hair, light touch, or even spontaneous movements of the animal elicited withdrawal reactions and occasionally, vocalizations and resistance. The hair over the hindquarters became matted and dirty in contrast to the hair over the rest of the body, which the cat kept groomed in a normal fashion.

Once established, this hyperesthetic state persisted as long as the cat lived—in one case, more than three years. One cat, which became the special pet of the animal caretaker, would purr with pleasure when its head, neck, and forequarters were stroked or scratched but would jump away and show its displeasure when touched elsewhere. This cat would waken from sleep if a fly lit on its fur over the hyperesthetic zone, and occasionally, after a jump from a table had apparently increased the local irritation, it was observed to walk a few steps on its forepaws while holding its hind legs in the air.

In a subsequent study at the University of British Columbia, Dr. Kennard tried injecting the colloidal aluminum cream at higher levels in the cat spinal cord. In five animals she injected an extremely small amount of the cream into the cord on its right lateral aspect in the midcervical region, while in three animals she administered the material intradurally at this level. The consequent hyperesthesia and hyperreflexia were greatest near the level of injection but also involved all of the body below this level. Transection of the cord in the thoracic region, far below the level of injection, did not abolish the hyperreflexia in the isolated segments, which indicated that their abnormal irritability was not directly dependent upon the presence of the originally affected cord segments. Postmortem examinations of the spinal cords showed some damage to large myelinated fibers in the vicinity of the injection and gave the impression that small cells with short fibers may have suffered still more damage, although the extent of this damage could not be ascertained. In her conclusions, Dr. Kennard stated: "The hyperalgesia cannot be attributed to potentiation of parts of the central nervous system rostral to the lesion since it persists following decerebration and following section of the cord both above and below the level of injection. The hyperalgesia must therefore be caused by the potentiation of neurones remaining active within the partially destroyed segmental systems of the cord. In this respect it resembles the conditions in man which may follow injuries to peripheral nerves." (Kennard 1953)

This is an important contribution but it seems to me that it still leaves us in doubt as to the ultimate nature of nerve "irritation." Even if we assume that its primary effect is on the nerve cells directly affected by its presence, this would not explain why its effects had spread to involve reflex circuits at a distance. The primary lesion in causalgia is an injury to a peripheral nerve fiber, yet the characteristic feature of this syndrome is the central perturbation of function. The primary injury to the motor cortex due to freezing or the alumina ion directly involves only the outer layer of cortical cells, yet the Jacksonian seizures are obviously attributable to dysfunction in distant nerve circuits. And the persistence of a hyperreflexia in isolated segments of the spinal cord, far from the site of the injection at cervical levels, seems to raise similar questions. It seems to me that such questions may prove more difficult to answer than why a female dog's rectus muscle reflex reverses itself when she becomes pregnant.

Midbrain Lesions and "Zombies"

When Morruzzi and Magoun reported their discovery of the RAS in the midbrain RF, some investigators wondered why such a massive lesion was used to demonstrate its presence. Previous studies had indicated that much more restricted lesions of the RF had altered animal behavior. For example, a few years earlier Bailey and Davis had put a copper wire through a cat's aqueduct of Sylvius and had passed an electrical current through it to burn out the collar of central gray matter around it (Bailey and Davis 1944). Cats that had this localized lesion were thereafter curiously inert and aphonic, a condition called "akinetic mutism." We had also observed that while we were making lesions in this region we sometimes hit a point that elicited a loud "meow" even though the cat was deeply asleep under a general anesthetic. This single vocalization was a sort of "swan song" for the animal because it never was heard to vocalize thereafter no matter how long the cat survived after the operation.

With such observations in mind, we wished to see what effects could be produced on a cat's behavior when lesions were made in the RF that spared the central gray matter. So, Fred Johnson prepared a few cats with these more restricted lesions in the RF. For a few days after the operation, these animals remained in a semicomatose condition. Then, it was possible to rouse them to a limited amount of activity. That they had awakened was indicated by their spontaneous movements and by the replacement of sleep waves by the desynchronized activity that is characteristic of the conscious brain. Yet these cats were far from normal in their behavior. They paid little or no attention to loud sounds, bright lights, noxious stimuli, or a threat of attack by a barking dog. Sensory stimuli seemed to have lost their meaning to the animals so that they failed to react to situations that would have greatly excited a normal cat. When moving about a room they would sometimes avoid obstacles as if they saw them, and had deliberately avoided them, while at other times they would run into the obstacles as if totally blind. Such a cat might sit on a table looking around the room as if aware of its situation and then would walk off the table edge and fall to the floor with a thud, while making no effort to right itself during the fall. At times, it failed to notice when someone stood on its tail, at other times it might look around vaguely and pull slowly away from the restraint but it never vocalized, bared its claws, or otherwise behaved as if it was experiencing any pain. These cats had to be tube fed because they would not swallow meat put in their mouths nor would they lap up milk after their heads had been dipped in it. In fact, they would not even lick off cream from around their mouths. They never groomed themselves or evinced the slightest interest in their welfare.

In short, these cats with the limited RF lesions of the midbrain behaved like "zombies"—the living dead—whose mind and spirit had departed, leaving only an automaton to imitate the casual movements of life. The complete absence of the usual defensive responses to noxious stimuli made us wonder if these cats were capable of perceiving pain. The fact that they occasionally pulled away when someone stepped on their tails might suggest that they could still feel pain, but if so, their behavior indicated that they "just didn't give a damn." Such observations made us wonder if perhaps a still more localized lesion might abolish all pain perceptions without making a "zombie" of the experimental animal. But, as our subsequent studies will show, there is good reason to doubt that a "specific" pain pathway will ever be demonstrated in that cat brain.

21

Tracing Tooth-Pulp Responses into the Cat Brain

From the time the pain project was first organized, one of our principal objectives was to work out an experimental method that might enable us to trace the path, or paths, by which the pain "signal" reached the higher centers in the brain. Our plan was to use a single electrical pulse to stimulate some well-known pain source and then try to follow the responses to their ultimate destinations in the brain of an anesthetized cat. Once a path had been located we intended to implant an electrode in it so that we could activate this tract selectively when the cat was not under the influence of an anesthetic drug. The cat's behavior during this stimulation might show us whether this tract was related to pain perception. We felt that if we knew more about the neural substrates for this sensation we could try any number of experiments, such as finding out where and how anesthetic and analgesic drugs modified the signal pattern. We even hoped that our studies might provide some clues as to the nature of the perceptual process, as pain perception is blocked in a state of "analgesia" before other sensory perceptions are seriously impaired.

We knew before we started this endeavor that we were up against a most difficult problem and we were assured by experts that our efforts were almost certain to fail. The reasons for the pessimism included the following points. What is called "slow pain" is said to be carried by very small, nonmyelinated C fibers. These fibers are difficult to activate selectively because an electrical pulse of sufficient duration to elicit a response also activates all the nearby larger sensory fibers and the much greater amplitude of their responses obscures the C-fiber response.

Even if we could find a way to activate C fibers selectively it would be difficult to trace their slow-traveling, low-amplitude responses into the brain because the constant spontaneous activity in the brain would almost certainly obscure them. What is called "fast pain" is ascribed to activity in the smaller of the myelinated fibers of the A group. It would be difficult to work with this group of fibers because no one knew how to activate them selectively, nor could we be sure that they subserved pain and no other sensations. The experts did not doubt our ability to map out the course followed by responses to noxious stimuli within the brain; what they questioned was our ability to prove that these responses exclusively subserved pain. They felt that the main roadblock to progress in our investigation was our own basic assumption that nothing could properly be called pain unless it could be consciously perceived as such. The question they were asking was: "How do you expect to identify the neural substrates for this particular sensory experience when no one knows where or how a brain translates any "sensation" into a "perception"?

Whatever success we have had in overcoming these obstacles can be largely attributed to two factors. The first was that our pain research team had its own skills, supplemented by those of a brilliant group of young neurophysiologists who joined us for periods ranging from six months to three years. The second factor was our choice of the tooth as the site for stimulation. We found that the teeth of cats as well as of humans are exclusively supplied by small myelinated fibers of the A group, in what is referred to as the "delta-gamma elevation" or the "delta pile." These fibers all have undifferentiated, "naked" terminals distributed in the dentin of a tooth and derive from nerve cells in the spinal root of the trigeminal nerve. The fibers from these nerve cells range from 1 to 7 microns in diameter, with an average of about 3 microns, and they conduct nerve impulses at rates from 30 to 45 meters per second with an average rate of 33 meters per second. They can be activated by a single electrical pulse of 0.06 milliseconds' duration. The strength-duration curve for these fibers in a cat's tooth is approximately the same as the strength-duration curve for the sensory fibers supplied to human teeth. Neither of these curves is similar to the S-D curves for either C fibers or the larger myelinated fibers of the A group. When the sensory fibers in a cat's tooth are activated they produce a response of such good amplitude that it is not difficult to follow along the classical sensory pathway to the relay nuclei of the thalamus and from there to the sensory area of the cerebral cortex. It is true that there are a few small nonmyelinated fibers to be found in the tooth pulp but they apparently represent vasomotor units supplied to blood vessels rather than sensory fibers; at least, we were never able to demonstrate that C fibers make any contribution to pain from a tooth. These more-or-less technical generalizations can be interpreted as meaning that the tooth is an ideal site for stimulation because it is supplied by a particular class of sensory fiber with known physiological properties, among which is the ability to transmit "sensations" that are "perceived" as pain. In other words, we would be dealing with what has been called "fast pain."

The story behind these generalizations was not simple. In our first experiments we simply bored two holes into the root canal of an anesthetized cat's tooth and sent in a single, square-wave pulse of sufficient voltage to activate its intrinsic sensory fibers. In a lightly anesthetized animal each single pulse elicited a reflex twitch of the lower jaw, so that we could be sure that the sensory barrage was at least reaching the spinal nucleus of the fifth nerve in the cat's brainstem. When we inserted a pick-up electrode into this root we were surprised at the ease with which we could record a response of considerable magnitude. The typical response was a double wave, the first wave being fast, sharp, and smooth, the second being more irregular and prolonged. It was possible to demonstrate that the first wave registered the response in the fiber, while the second one was created by the firing of secondary neurons in the spinal nucleus. This nuclear discharge was of such high amplitude that we felt we would have no serious difficulty following the response upward in the brain.

The thing that disturbed us about these observations was that the responses we elicited from the tooth were obviously not carried by C fibers. We had rather naively assumed that "toothache" was subserved by C fibers, an assumption that many other investigators seemed to share—notably, the medical director of the foundation that was supporting our research. The responses we were recording had an amplitude that was perhaps a hundred times greater than would be generated by C fibers, their latency was very much shorter, and the duration of the pulse we used to elicit the responses was approximately one-tenth of the pulse width required to activate C fibers. Then we discovered that when we applied the same short-pulse stimulus to one of our own amalgam-filled teeth, we experienced first, at liminal voltages, a faint "tap" that seemed to come from deep in the tooth and then, as the voltage was increased, a faint pricking sensation. High-voltage pulses caused sharp, well-localized pain. Based on these observations we decided it might be wise to see what the anatomists and dentists knew about the intrinsic nerve supply to the tooth and how a tooth develops from the dental lamina. A review of the literature did not settle the C-fiber question. The consensus seemed to be that most of the intrinsic sensory fibers to the tooth were small myelinated fibers of the A group, although several investigators were still searching for C fibers as the source for pain from a tooth. The literature also called our attention to the rich plexus of sensory fibers in the periodontal membrane, and it seemed possible that the pulse we were using was of sufficient intensity to activate these extrinsic fibers so that they might create the responses we were recording. We would have to rule out this possibility before we could go further with our investigation.

To solve this problem we tried every method we could devise to insulate the tooth from surrounding tissues so as to make sure that our stimuli acted only on sensory fibers intrinsic to the tooth itself, but technical difficulties prevented us from reaching any final answer. The solution was partly a matter of luck and partly due to a better understanding of how a tooth develops. One day in January 1951, we were preparing to make one last effort to insulate a cat's canine tooth from its surrounding tissues. When we went to the animal room no adult cats were available. Instead, we were offered a kitten that had just lost its milk teeth and whose permanent teeth were not fully erupted. We were reluctant to accept this animal because its canine teeth were so small. We were sure we would have difficulty placing our electrodes in the tooth pulp, but we also knew that a tooth begins its dentin deposit at its outer limits and then it progresses inwardly before it reaches its final form with a cap of enamel and a narrow pulp cavity. Sure enough, when we dissected out this kitten's canine tooth we found a thin shell of dentin within which was a worm-like mass of pulp substance. This mass was highly vascular but quite tough, so that it was not difficult to dissect it free from the dentin shell, except at its proximal attachment. We laid this elongated mass on some insulating material and inserted two insect needle electrodes into its distal end. When we stimulated the mass through these needles we were able to pick up responses in the nerve root that were similar in all respects to those we had been recording in adult cats. After carefully measuring the latency of these responses we reversed the process by stimulating centrally and picking up the response in the tooth pulp. The latency of this antidromic response was exactly the same as the latency of the orthodromic response, which implied that the same fibers were involved in both cases. Given that the antidromic response was carried by fibers intrinsic to the tooth pulp we felt this supported our assumption that the responses we had been recording in the nerve root in our former experiments originated in the tooth itself.

Once we felt reasonably sure that our stimulating pulses were activating sensory fibers intrinsic to the tooth, we had no serious difficulty in tracing the responses all the way up to the face area of the sensory cortex. That is, we had no difficulty tracing the responses in one particular pathway that crossed the brainstem and skirted the midbrain RF to reach the relay nuclei of the thalamus and from there to the cortex. The response in this pathway was always fast, sharply defined, and of high amplitude no matter what the depth of the anesthesia. This apparently was the classical "three-neuron pain pathway" we had learned to diagram in medical school, but was this the only pathway by which the tooth-pulp-induced responses could reach higher levels in the brain? To answer this question we began a systematic millimeter-by-millimeter exploration across the midbrain, searching with our recording electrodes for responses to tooth-pulp stimulation. In doing so we picked up definite responses in quite unexpected situations. For example, we often recorded responses deep in the RF, particularly if the animal was lightly anesthetized. We had no explanation to offer for these findings until Moruzzi and Magoun reported their discovery of the reticular activating system traversing the midbrain reticular formation. We then were apprised of the supreme importance of making our explorations in the unanesthetized brain if we wanted to learn more about the nature of "pain" as we defined it. We found this task to be enormously difficult. Anyone wishing to know more about the technical aspects of our investigations and the impressions we derived from it must read the published reports. But here I am trying to avoid technical language and I shall refer only to five areas in the midbrain of interest to us. I have designated them only by numbers and have indicated their approxi-

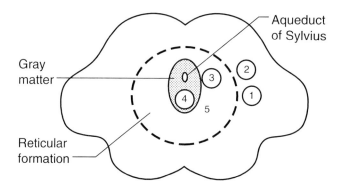

Fig. 1. This diagrammatic cross-section of the cat brain through the midbrain shows the reticular formation (5, within dotted circle) containing the aqueduct of Sylvius and its surrounding gray matter. The numbers refer to areas where additional electrical responses were recorded following tooth-pulp stimulation. Tracts in the vicinity of (1) are part of the classical three-neuron sensory system to cortex. Those near (2) correspond to the pain and temperature pathway to thalamus. Those near (3) produce consistent hyperesthesia. Area 4 is the central gray matter and cats with lesions here are less responsive to noxious stimulation. Cats learned to avoid electrical stimulation at (2) and (4) by pressing a lever.

mate location in a crude diagram of a cross-section of the cat brain through the midbrain (Fig. 1). From each of the five areas we could consistently record responses to tooth-pulp stimulation in the unanesthetized brain but the responses recorded in different areas were never exactly alike in latency, amplitude, and susceptibility to the influence of anesthetic drugs. The area roughly delimited by the dotted circle represents the reticular formation in the center of which is the aqueduct of Sylvius and its surrounding gray matter. Areas 1 and 2 are outside the RF and are part of the "classical" sensory systems which, together with the classical motor tracts, form a huge collar around the RF.

In area 1 we *always* could record a response to a single electrical pulse applied to a tooth in the contralateral jaw. The response was fast, sharp, and of high amplitude no matter how we might try to depress it with analgesic or anesthetic drugs. The responses passing through this tract could be traced to the relay nuclei of the thalamus and from there to the face area of the cat's sensory cortex. One might say that here was the classic example of a "three-neuron pain pathway" because it carries nerve impulses from a known pain source to the sensory cortex. Nevertheless, these impulses evidently are sufficient to produce pain perceptions because they are not blocked by the deepest states of unconsciousness.

In area 2 the responses to tooth stimulation were slightly longer in latency and considerably smaller in amplitude. Although they were stronger on the contralateral side we sometimes could pick them up ipsilaterally. Their amplitude could be reduced by giving the animal a few inhalations of nitrous oxide gas or ether, a fact that enabled us to distinguish them from the responses over tract 1 to the face area of the sensory cortex. This fact also helped in following the responses in this tract to the posterior part of the thalamus and from there to both the first and second sensory areas bilaterally. We had the impression that area 2 represented the trigeminal portion of the so-called "pain and temperature tract."

From areas 3 and 4 we consistently picked up responses to tooth stimulation and with less consistency from the RF in the general region of 5. The responses were stronger on the contralateral side but could always be recorded bilaterally. They had a considerably longer latency and a much lower amplitude than those recorded in areas 1 and 2. A few breaths of nitrous oxide gas or ether reduced the size of the responses to about half their previous size in areas 3 and 4 and often wiped out the response in area 5.

These and related observations gave us the impression that conduction in tract 1 was not the source for pain perception and that impulses ascending bilaterally in areas 3, 4, and 5 to distant parts of the brain might have as much, or more, to do with pain perception than those carried by the classical "pain and temperature" tract. To test the validity of these assumptions we devised three sets of experiments, which I can describe very briefly.

Destructive Lesions in Midbrain Areas

Our plan in this experiment was to selectively block conduction in tract 2, 3, or 4 in cats and to subsequently test their reactions to heat and pinprick stimulation. It was necessary to operate on many cats before the tests could be started because the small size of a cat's midbrain makes it almost impossible to place a lesion so accurately that it affects but one of these exceedingly tiny areas. This tends to make the tests "blind" because we would not be able to tell just where the lesion had been placed in a particular cat until its midbrain had been examined microscopically after the tests had been run. The tests were done in a cage with two compartments separated only by a barrier four inches high. The floor of one compartment was constructed so that the experimenter could stimulate the cat's feet with either heat or pinprick by remote control. All the animal had to do to escape from such stimuli was to hop over the low barrier. Each of the seventy-nine cats used in this experiment was subjected to a series of tests in this cage each day for five days and their reaction time was recorded for each trial. At the end of this test series the cats were sacrificed and their midbrains were sectioned to see how accurately the single lesion had been placed. Only then could we analyze our data, that is, could see if there were any correlation between the site of a midbrain lesion and the animal's behavior in relation to noxious stimuli.

The results of this experiment were not as conclusive as we might have wished because there were only six cats with bilateral lesions satisfactorily localized in area 2; five cats with lesions involving only area 4 bilaterally; and six cats with bilateral lesions localized to area 3. However, our data seemed to justify the following generalizations: Cats with lesions in either areas 2 or 4 seemed definitely more impervious to noxious stimulation than were our controls. Cats with lesions in area 2 seemed much less sensitive to prick stimuli than to heat and this loss of sensibility did not seem to be altered during the five days of testing. The cats with lesions in area 4 seemed less sensitive to both forms of stimulation than did the controls and less sensitive to heat stimuli than to pricking. One cat with this lesion sat placidly on hot wires and the experimenter noted an odor of singed hair before the cat moved across the barrier. But this happened only on the first day of testing and by the fifth day its reaction time seemed more nearly normal. Cats with bilateral lesions in area 3 behaved as if they had been *hypersensitized* to both forms of stimulation. This observation was quite unexpected because we are sure that the responses we had been recording from the tooth in this area were ascending to higher brain levels. There is a possibility that this same area also contained a descending tract that normally served to inhibit impulse patterns contributing to pain perceptions. Whatever the explanation may be, five of the six cats in this group were definitely more sensitive than normal to both prick and heat stimuli. There seemed to be an excessive "urgency" in their immediate response to pinprick, often yowling, leaping high in the air, and "somersaulting" across the barrier. They seemed to dislike being handled, walked about gingerly, often flicking one paw after the other as if to rid them of some persistent irritation. One of these cats, when its paws were pricked, would yowl and leap for the mesh at the top of the cage and then would cling to it upside down in crossing the barrier.

Implanted Electrodes

In each of eight cats, two electrodes were permanently implanted in the midbrain. One was placed to stimulate selectively the anterolateral aspect of the central gray matter (near area 4) and the other was placed in the region of area 2. Each cat was trained to press a lever to terminate a train of electrical stimuli applied to one of three areas: the "pain tract" (area 2), the central gray (area 4), or its feet, by way of the grid on which it was standing. By varying the order in which these three noxious stimuli were used in testing, we hoped to be able to decide how much each cat was able to "generalize" from one form of stimulation to another. For example, two cats received the shock to their feet first and when they had learned that pressing the lever terminated the stimuli, they were next trained to press the lever to avoid shocks to the pain tract (area 2) and finally to the central gray (area 4). The next pair of cats received their noxious stimuli in a different order—central, lateral, and peripheral—and so on. The recorded results of this experiment gave no definite evidence that any of these cats had "generalized" from one test situation to the other, although there was no doubt that they all "disliked" all three forms of stimulation and learned quite quickly how to avoid them. In another experiment with this same set of cats, each animal had two levers it could press, one that would shut off a stimulus applied to area 4 and another that terminated a train of shocks to area 2. None of these cats seemed to have any difficulty in learning which lever controlled which sensory input centrally. In other words, the cats *seemed able to distinguish the perceptual effects of one tract activation from the other and both were apparently obnoxious.*

Editor's Note: In Dr. Livingston's original manuscript this chapter concluded with a paragraph under the heading "Central Gray Matter Stimulation in the Monkey." It has been placed in Appendix C because it is primarily a methodological description and the result is not quantifiable.

Comment

These experiments do not tell us where or how pain is perceived in the brain but they do argue against the idea that the essential area is the sensory cortex and that analgesic states are directly attributable to a depression of function in these particular cortical cells. They argue against any notion that pain is packaged within a "pain and temperature tract." They also seem to reduce the chances that anyone will ever find a single specific pathway for pain. At least we can be sure that it can never be demonstrated in the anesthetized brain.

22

The Functional Organization
of the Central Nervous System

Over the years, all of William F. Allen's predictions as to the important functions performed by the reticular formation have been substantiated by experimental observations. As we followed this work we found ourselves thinking less and less in terms of unitary specificity and more and more in terms of "pattern," less in terms of mechanism and more in terms of "ongoing transactions." This interpretive trend was augmented by seminar discussions of the ideas of such great men as Erwin Schrödinger, George Coghill, Judson Herrick, Percy Bridgman, Adelbert Ames, and Karl Lashley. To illustrate the trend of our thinking, here is a synopsis of a seminar discussion that opened with a review of the work of George Coghill.

As a young man Coghill studied for the ministry, but he quit in the midst of his training because he could not endure the intolerance and dogmatism of the fundamentalist instruction he was receiving. He was in a state of mental turmoil and uncertainty as to his future when he went on a camping trip in New Mexico. While there he had the good fortune to meet Clarence Herrick,[1] the newly appointed president of the University of New Mexico. Coghill confided to Herrick that his greatest interest in life was to find out more about how the brain functions and its relationship to behavior and mental processes. Herrick encouraged him to study zoology and to undertake an intensive study of mind-brain relationships in some of the simpler forms of animal life. He offered the facilities of his laboratory to the young man and started

---

[1]*Editor's Note:* This is C.L. Herrick, the elder brother of C. Judson Herrick.

him on his long career as an investigator in 1897, the same year that Hughlings Jackson was announcing his "doctrine of levels."

Coghill's first teaching assignment began in 1906 at Pacific University in Forest Grove, Oregon. He found little zoological teaching material there but the streams and ponds in the vicinity abounded with *Ambystoma*, a common species of salamander. He used these little animals in his zoology classes and made them the focus of his investigations over the next forty years. His objective was to establish some correlation between the development of the brain in very young salamanders and the elaboration of their behavioral patterns. He began his investigations with a careful study of the embryonic brain and the exact time at which its motor and sensory connections with the skin and skeletal muscles were established. He found that the motor systems were clearly established at an early stage in the animal's development. The sensory systems developed later, the central parts of the specific sensory systems being organized before their peripheral connections had been completed. Interposed between the motor and sensory components of the *Ambystoma* brain was a massive collection of small nerve cells that Coghill called the "neuropil." This structure appeared in the brain at an early developmental stage as a felt-work of nerve cells with no long processes but many intercommunicating branches.

Coghill began his investigations without any preconceived ideas as to how a nervous system might function. He was inclined to accept the teachings of Hughlings Jackson that the "simple reflex arc" was the functional unit from which the entire system was built up and that voluntary movement is little more than "a glorified reflex." Coghill was willing to accept this hypothesis but he wished to test it for himself. However, when he tested his developing salamander embryos for their response to stimulation he was unable to demonstrate a single "simple reflex." On the contrary, the first response of the skeletal muscles to skin stimulation was a "total response" that involved a contraction of all the muscles that had any connection with the central nervous system. As the more caudally situated muscles developed their innervation, the stimulus produced a strong body flexion that overlapped the head and tail; later, the more rapid transmission of the excitation resulted in "S" contractions in wave-like progressions that produced swimming movements.

Coghill usually worked at a large, round table, the top of which could be rotated. At the margin of the tabletop was a continuous row of petri dishes, each containing a single embryo; all the embryos in the row were derived from the same clutch of eggs and were at exactly the same stage of development. He and his assistant sat opposite each other at this table and used a stiff hair to stimulate each animal on a particular skin area and then record the muscular response in relation to the exact age of each embryo. These tests went on hour after hour, once for seventy-two hours in succession. Thousands of such observations convinced Coghill that the basic organization of the central nervous system was motor and its primary function was to produce total body movements. As he followed the later development of these animals after their limbs had developed, he found that any stimulation produced coordinated swimming movements long before the individual limbs could be moved; that the proximal joints of limbs were moved before the more distal ones, and that purposeful movements appeared last of all. From its behavior, it was evident that the young salamander learned to satisfy its primitive needs by experience derived from action. It was Coghill's impression that the animal "learned by doing" how to suppress the inappropriate parts of the total response to the environmental stimulus and thus to "individuate" a purposeful movement. He conceived the idea that "action" and "experience" gradually served to emancipate parts of the total pattern from its original dominance, so that the total response pattern could be suppressed except under conditions of extreme stress or massive stimulation.

As he watched a salamander's progressive improvement in performance, it seemed that the animal was developing a low-grade type of "intelligence," as if it had stored its sensory experiences in some way so that these memories could serve as a guide for future behavior. He believed that the neuropil was the structure in which this learning process must take place, perhaps by some kind of growth change of the nerve cell connections. He believed that the sensory input diffused out over this network of cells before reaching the motor systems. At first the motor response was massive and unselective, but as the incoming time-space patterns were constantly repeated, some growth change in the neuropil tended to fix them there. As the animal tried to satisfy its body needs the response to a particular sensory input became less diffuse and better channeled for effective behavior.

Coghill's denial that action patterns are built up from simple reflexes prompted a controversy that has been slow to subside. Yet, his deviation from the orthodox interpretations of his day went much deeper than this. He could not visualize the nervous system as a mere aggregate of specialized end stations connected with one another in a simple sequence by the long-fiber tracts. Rather, he saw it as a functional whole, possessed of a growth potential within a diffusion system interposed between the sensory and motor components and constantly playing its influence on both input and output. In 1929 he wrote: "Conduction, however complex the organization may be, cannot fully account for the role of the nervous system in behavior. The conventional figures of the telephone with its switchboards to illustrate how the nervous system works is totally inadequate unless the inventor and the operator be included in the figure. In the nervous system the growth potential is at once the inventor and the operator" (Coghill 1929).

Coghill's failure to demonstrate simple reflexes in the salamander and his assignment of such functions as "mentation" and individuation to what appeared to be a simple network of nerve cells did not make him popular among his contemporaries. The prevailing view at that time was that the mental capacities of a brain were functions of its cerebral cortex, but salamanders have no cortex. Was Coghill implying that these stupid little animals can "think"? What evidence was there that the human brain contains a simple polysynaptic diffusion system comparable to a "neuropil" and possessed with the capacity to modulate behavior based on experience? Surely, this capacity must demand more highly organized brain structures than a salamander possesses. How could Coghill ever expect to account for the activities of such a complex functional whole as the human brain without first analyzing the functions of each of its component parts?

In the fascinating dialogues that Judson Herrick has recorded between himself and Coghill, they seem to be turning this last question back on their critics by asking, "How can you expect to understand the functional capacities of the human brain unless you first identify the source of the most primitive capacity for storage and recall? Any animal that can learn to respond to environmental cues with changes in behavior better suited to its primary needs and purposes must be able to receive and store sensory input and then be able to use this stored information as a guide to future behavior" (Herrick 1956).

In recent years many scientists seem to be adopting this same line of reasoning and in their search for the "where and how" of storage as the source of adaptive behavior they have moved down the scale of animal life from the mammals to such invertebrates as the squid and the octopus, to such insects as the cockroach, and even to flukes and clams, whose total nervous system consists of only a few thousand individual nerve cells. Horridge has shown that the ventral cord of a decapitated cockroach exhibits some degree of adaptive behavior (Horridge 1962), and more recently Cohen has demonstrated that adaptive behavior can be "learned" by even so simple a nerve net as exists in a single isolated cockroach ganglion. He found that when the leg innervated by this ganglion comes in contact with a pool of acid, the leg is withdrawn and, as the acid level is raised, the leg muscles again alter the limb posture to keep it out of the acid (Eisenstein and Cohen 1965).

As we reviewed these many investigations and discussed the theories offered to account for storage and recall, it seemed to us that Coghill had given us a new concept of neural function. At least we were acquiring a greater respect for the functional capacities of the reticular formation. It was easier for us to understand how the great masses of reticular cells in the brainstem could modulate both the sensory input and the motor output to maintain the organism in harmony with its internal and external environments. However, our attention to the reticular formation was not confined to its brainstem portion for it seemed likely that it extended upward to all the higher brain levels as well as down the entire length of the spinal cord. We no longer could regard the spinal portion as being merely a few scattered nerve cells left behind during phylogenetic development but as an essential part of an integrative whole. The concept of the "internuncial pool" had helped us get away from the restrictive influence of the "simple reflex arc" account of cord function but we still tended to think of these pools as being segmentally independent. Now we could understand how the reticular cells might harmonize their activities and perhaps could serve as the agency by which dysfunction in neuron pools at one level might spread to other levels. As our respect for the integrative powers of the reticular formation increased we could see how it might serve to weld the central nervous system into a functional whole.

We tried to construct a diagram that would depict this exciting concept of functional unity but the "doctrine of levels" seemed to be so ingrained in our thinking that most of our diagrams ended up looking

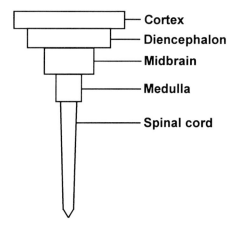

Fig. 1. The "doctrine of levels" attempted to compartmentalize various functions of the central nervous system in a hierarchically organized series of anatomic units.

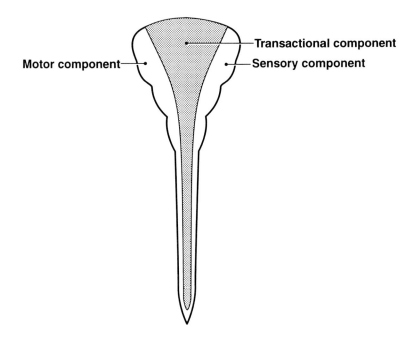

Fig. 2. The functional attributes of the central nervous system may be better explained and investigated by admitting the possibility that they consist of "transactions" occurring at many levels of the brain and spinal cord. Such transactions may be initiated by sensory input and always find their expression in motor activity but have an identity of their own that is greater than the sum of these two parts.

too much like the drawing in Fig. 1. Finally, we came up with a diagram (Fig. 2) showing the sensory and motor systems separated by a "transactional" component through which all sensory input must diffuse to reach the motor systems. The indentations along the margins of this figure were intended to suggest, but not to emphasize, the segmental arrangement.

We preferred to label the interposed system of neurons the "transactional" component rather than calling it a "neuropil" because this latter term is often used too restrictively to convey any idea of the dynamic plasticity we attributed to this part of the nervous system. We did not visualize it as an amorphous mass of undifferentiated nerve cells through which impulses passed in a haphazard fashion. It is conceivable that in the very young infant the cells making up this functional unit might be unorganized in the same way that embryonic blood vessels are first represented as a vast syncytium of capillaries, and where only later does a selective channeling occur to enlarge a few of them to form arteries and veins. This simile suggests something of the way in which, based on experience, reiterated patterns of sensory impulses might become channeled so that the motor response is appropriate to the stimulus. Nor could we think of this functional unit as representing merely vestiges of some primitive cell type from which the specialized centers and long tracts have developed during phylogenetic evolution. Instead we regarded the "transactional" component as being an essential part of every nervous system, from the most primitive to the most complex.

The ability to profit from past experience in determining purposive behavior is a distinguishing characteristic animals. In general, the more complex an animal's brain, the more diversified its behavior and the more discriminating its response to environmental demands. An animal is built for action so it is to be expected that the motor components of its nervous system should be dominant in its structural and functional organization. Next, the animal needs a sensory component to maintain contact with its environment. Yet, if these two were the only components of its brain, the animal would be little more than an automaton. There must be another functional unit linking them, otherwise the sensory input would never acquire any meaning and the motor output would never serve any purposive value to the animal.

It was our opinion that the brainstem reticular formation constituted an essential transactional component of the nervous system. We did not believe that it was necessary to assume that it was the most important part of this interposed unit. Instead, we tended to visualize it as including the association areas of the cerebral cortex, the limbic system, and perhaps other parts of the brain as well as the reticular formation and the internuncial pools throughout the neuraxis.

23

Habituation

I once stalled my car in a snowdrift and was given a lift into town by an elderly neighbor driving an open, Model-T Ford. The car was in an advanced stage of dissolution and as it rattled and swayed along I expected that at any moment it might lie down in the middle of the road. The old man did little talking and I could see that he was obviously worried about something. I assumed that he was worried about the increasing force of the storm until I noticed that he was leaning forward over the wheels with his head cocked to one side, as if listening to something. I asked him the cause for his concern and he replied, "She ain't running right, Doc. That loud sound you hear just come this morning but I just can't seem to place it!" When I admitted that I didn't know which particular sound he was referring to, he tried to point it out to me by saying, "It's right down thar somewheres going 'chuck-a-lug-chuck-a-lug' all the time and getting louder and louder. Can't you hear it, Doc? It's just as plain." Only then did I realize that he had long since identified the source of all the customary creaks and rattles in the old car, so that he was no longer hearing them and could give his entire attention to the new sound. I was probably hearing it too, but I was too distracted by the many other rattles to pick it out, although it was evidently clearly audible to him.

It is easier to think of other similar examples of "habituation"—that ability of a person to disregard sensory signals coming from a familiar environment so as to permit focusing his attention on signals that have more immediate significance because they relate to his needs and purposes. Perhaps the simplest example of habituation is that of

189

the child who is so familiar with his mother's voice and who has become so engrossed in reading a comic book that he fails to respond to repeated calls to come to supper. Only when she comes to take the book away and scold him for not answering does he show signs of having normal hearing. When she demands to know why he failed to respond to her calls he insists that he did not hear them. She is equally insistent that he must have heard them because she had shouted loud enough to have been heard a block away. She thinks the boy deliberately ignored her calls because it seems inconceivable that sounds of that intensity could have failed to register in his consciousness.

Country folk who visit in a city complain that they are kept awake at night by the sounds of traffic, while city dwellers find the absence of night noises in the country disquieting. But both people and animals soon adjust themselves to the sounds of any new environment. With training, people discover that they can maintain a considerable degree of auditory selectiveness even during sleep. The classical example of this was the Chicago housewife whose apartment was close to the elevated railway tracks and who could sleep soundly while the trains roared by, yet was immediately awakened by the faint cry of her baby.

This sensory selectivity applies to all our special senses and can be developed to a high degree. Most of us make no special effort to cultivate this selective capacity so that we are amazed by the discriminatory powers of experts whether they are wine tasters, naturalists, wool buyers, physicians, or aborigine trackers. These persons have learned what to look for and to disregard irrelevancies so they can scan complex problems for their significance and reach conclusions with a speed and accuracy that seem uncanny. Yet all of us acquire this sensory selectivity to some degree without any conscious effort. In fact, there is ample experimental evidence to indicate that our brains constantly exert a regulatory control over all sensory input in accordance with our bodily needs and our purposes. Practically all this evidence has been gathered within the last ten years and many important investigations are still under way. However, my limited knowledge of this field is confined to the studies of brain mechanisms regulating auditory input, so I can give only a brief report of this part of the story. My first contact with these investigations came during a visit to Herbert Jasper's neurophysiology laboratory in Montreal and I think the year was 1954.

Among the many interesting things that Herb showed me during that visit was an experiment he and Sharpless were conducting (Sharpless 1956). In a soundproof box they had placed a cat with an electrode attached to its skull so that its recording tip was directly over the cat's auditory cortex. A fine wire cable, which did not restrict the cat's movements within the box, led from the electrode to a plug in the top of the box. By connecting this plug to an oscilloscope the experimenters could visualize the changes in electrical activity in the cat's auditory cortex at any time they wished. Within the box a tone of fixed pitch and intensity sounded at intervals hour after hour and day after day. For a long time after the cat had been exposed to this reiterated tone, the recordings showed that an auditory response of considerable magnitude was reaching this part of the cortex each time the tone sounded. However, after hours or days of exposure to this same tone, the amplitude of the response diminished until there was almost no evidence that the sensory impulses were activating cortical cells. That this disappearance of the cortical response was not due to "fatigue" of the cortical cells could be demonstrated by altering the pitch or the intensity of the tone, after which the cortical responses again appeared in full amplitude. However, if the reiterated tone remained identical the cortical responses never reappeared. The cat was said to have become "habituated" to that particular sound.

In themselves, these observations are not surprising because they accord so well with our own experiences in which we fail to "hear" sounds to which we have become accustomed. The usual explanation offered to account for this failure to perceive sounds is the same one that we have proposed before as the orthodox interpretation of the phenomenon in which perceptions of pain are not directly proportional to stimulus intensity: "The sensation of pain remains unchanged and only the individual's 'reaction' to it is altered." However, the observations of the habituated cat suggest that this interpretation might be tested experimentally. Of course, the cat can never tell us whether it is still hearing the tone, but we might get some information on this point if we could find out the level in the nervous system at which the auditory responses are being blocked before they can reach the cortex. At least, we might get information as to whether the blockade was "psychological" or due to some more fundamental brain process.

Raul Hernández-Peón, who had worked with our pain project team for a year, was one of the neurophysiologists who followed up this lead and I shall confine my comments to his observations (Hernández-Peón et al. 1956). He first implanted a recording electrode in the cochlear nucleus of a cat and then repeated the experiment that Jasper and Sharpless had performed. His aim was to find out whether the auditory responses were getting through this first relay station from the ear. His first discovery was that before the cat had become habituated to the reiterated tone or click the responses were ascending in a normal fashion all the way to the auditory cortex; a temporary suppression of the response occurred whenever the cat's attention was diverted. For example, when the cat was presented with two mice in a glass jar, the responses in both the cochlear nucleus and at the cortex were markedly diminished as long as the cat's attention appeared to be focused on the mice. As soon as the mice were taken away the responses returned to their previous amplitude, that is, until the cat had become habituated to the sound, after which the responses were again suppressed. The same things occurred when the odor of fish oil was blown into the cat's cage. As long as the cat was searching for the source of this appetizing odor the cochlear responses were suppressed, but when it ceased its search the responses returned to their original amplitude until habituation was established. These observations indicated that the mechanisms subserving attention could extend their influence far below any possible "perceptual" level, at least with regard to the cochlear nucleus. In other words, the temporary blockade of the responses could not be attributed to activities restricted to the high levels of brain function at which "psychological" processes have been assumed to occur.

Although it was still impossible to say that the cat "heard" nothing of the sound while its attention was being diverted, it was evident that its capacity to hear had been greatly reduced in this state and still further reduced or abolished after it had become habituated to the sound. Apparently, some inhibitory mechanism in the brain was blocking the sensory input at the first relay station. The next problem was to find out where this inhibitory influence originated. To solve it, Raul used cats that had already become habituated to the reiterated sound, that is, whose cochlear responses were being persistently suppressed. He found three ways to restore the responses promptly to their original amplitude, all three apparently involving the brainstem reticular formation. The first way was to make a lesion in this part of the formation; the second was to sever its connections with the cochlear nucleus; and the third was to put the cat deeply asleep under some anesthetic drug known to depress activity in the reticular formation. The interesting thing about this third method for restoring conduction to the auditory cortex was that as soon as the habituated cat awakened from its drugged sleep, the responses again failed to get past this first relay station from the ear.

Robert Galambos and his collaborators studied the auditory system in experimental animals for several years and made many important contributions to our understanding of this remarkable power of the brain to suppress portions of the sensory input at levels far below any possible perceptual level (Galambos 1959). In one set of experiments Galambos exposed a monkey to reiterated audible clicks until electrical responses completely habituated in the auditory cortex or any part of the brainstem in which he had planted additional electrodes. Then he "reinforced" the auditory stimulus by blowing a light puff of air across the monkey's face each time the click sounded. Immediately the auditory responses appeared at the cortex with their original amplitude, as well as in the brainstem reticular formation. When he used other types of reinforcing stimuli he observed that electrical activity could be recorded in distant parts of the brain that were previously inactive, particularly if the stimulus carried any possible threat of punishment that might create emotional states of excitement or fear.

Galambos was also able to record responses to auditory stimuli in single nerve cells in the auditory cortex of unanesthetized, unrestrained cats under a variety of test conditions. In these explorations he located cells that do not react to sounds unless the cat is paying attention to them. For example, he found units that were not activated by sounds to which auditory units usually respond, but if some unusual sound attracted the cat's attention, these otherwise unresponsive cells promptly responded. Among the unique sounds that activated these "attention" units were the experimenter's voice, squeaks of a toy mouse, and hissing and tapping sounds. In one instance, clicks from a loudspeaker failed to activate a particular unit until Galambos pretended to tap on the speaker box and thus directed the cat's attention to it.

Studies of auditory habituation have indicated that this brain function can be manipulated by conditioning experiments in much the same way as other forms of learning. In fact, habituation seems to represent what might be called a form of negative learning in that with training the brain acquires the ability to shut out portions of the sensory input that have no immediate significance while letting in those portions toward which the individual's attention is directed or that are of greater significance for survival. The ultimate source of this regulating influence on sensory input is not known. It may be that the reticular formation is merely the "policeman" carrying out the orders from some higher brain level. At least we know that the reticular formation is constantly exerting an influence on the sensory input and that this influence extends at least as far as the first relay station through which sensory impulses must pass to reach the brain. There is even evidence to suggest that this inhibitory influence may extend all the way out to the sensory receptors at the periphery.

The phenomenon of habituation can be demonstrated in sensory systems other than the auditory and in all forms of animal life, from man down to simple creatures that have no special sense organs and whose total nervous system consists of a simple nerve net. This suggests that habituation, like other forms of learning, is a manifestation of some fundamental property of nervous tissue. It implies that while the animal is learning to cope with a hazardous environment the sensory input traversing its neural circuits leaves some sort of "trace" that serves to identify particular patterns in terms of significance so that certain channels to the motor output can be opened or closed to improve the animal's efficiency in coping with that environment. Numerous theories have been advanced as to the nature of the "trace" but there seem to be objections to all. Whether the trace eventually proves to be morphological, chemical, or molecular, the investigations of such men as Karl Lashley and Roger Sperry make it clear that the trace is not confined to single cells or even to a single center but must involve many neural circuits in the form of a pattern (Lashley 1929; Sperry 1966).

This interpretation is further supported by recordings from electrodes permanently implanted in an animal's brain to record electrical activity during learning. These recordings reveal a sequence of events about like this: When the animal encounters some new situation, electrical changes are initiated in many parts of the brain other than the specific cortices. As this same experience is repeated many times the extent of the brain involvement narrows, as if the original pattern were being reduced to some simpler code for subsequent recall. If the experience proves to pose no threat to the animal and to have no immediate significance in relation to its bodily needs and purposes, the brain response may eventually become greatly attenuated or may disappear entirely. If now the nature of the experience is suddenly changed, as by adding some reinforcing stimulus, the widespread response in the brain again reappears in its original amplitude (Magoun 1963, chap. 7). If the new stimulus suggests punishment or otherwise generates emotional excitement, the brain responses increase in amplitude and spread to new areas of the brain that had not been activated by the original experience. These neural events closely parallel the changes in behavior displayed by the animal during such a conditioning sequence. Its behavior indicates that any new sensory experience commands the animal's full attention until it learns that this event is of no immediate significance in relation to its needs and purposes. Then, in the interests of economy of effort the sensory input can be damped down or completely suppressed, so as to free the higher centers of the brain for more important business. Only when the event is accompanied by some threat does the "startle" reaction reappear, so the animal gives its full attention to the event in order to decide how to deal with the threat.

Our own efforts to acquire some new motor skill is a learning process that apparently involves a similar train of neural events. In learning to play golf we are aware of a thousand things that must be watched—the position of the feet, the grip, the back swing, the pivot, the snap of the wrists, keeping the head down, etc., etc. With practice our awareness of these components of the swing fades and we can concentrate on the effort to hit the ball cleanly and in the line we want it to go. Each lie presents its own problems until we can deal with each one effectively, whether it involves sand, mud, obstacles, or side hills. If we make a profession of playing golf we may eventually reach a stage in which we can shut out extraneous stimuli and focus on each objective with singleness of purpose. We approach a championship match with supreme confidence that we have our game "in the groove." The crowd assembles and a respectful hush falls as we tee up for the first shot. The ball is at exactly the right height and distance and after a few impressive waggles of the club, we start the backswing. At the height of the swing the "reinforcing" stimulus is provided by a loud sneeze from directly behind us. This is a test of concentration and self-control that tends to separate the men from the boys.

This "Mr. Mitty" digression is only partly in fun. I have used it deliberately as a prelude to the statement of my conviction that behavioral studies more accurately indicate how the human mind operates than do studies of function in the brains of anesthetized animals. Teachings based on such studies have led to mechanistic interpretations; they have fostered the use of the telephone exchange as the model for a brain; they have overemphasized the importance of the classical sensory pathways and the specific cortices in sensory perception; they have encouraged us to identify such diverse sensory experiences as pain and touch with particular stimuli; they have led us to assume that all pains are measurable in terms of stimulus intensity; they have fostered an artificial distinction between sensation and perception; and, worst of all in my opinion, they have given future medical practitioners the notion that emotional states have no power to alter the sensation of pain but can only change the person's "reaction" to it. And if, on top of all that, these teachings give the medical student the impression that his first duty in evaluating a patient's complaints of pain is to distinguish clearly between his "real" pain and his "reactions" to it, then I foresee trouble ahead for both the future practitioner and his patient.

The studies of auditory habituation have been exciting because they have given us a new appreciation of the dynamic plasticity of the unanesthetized brain. They teach us what we already should have known from our own sensory experiences and observation of animal behavior—that pain is not always measurable in terms of stimulus intensity. Even if we are among those who insist on making a distinction between the physical sensation and its perceptions, we can no longer maintain that the "sensation" is constant in terms of stimulus intensity, because we now know that the brain has the power to suppress the sensory signal before it can ascend to the brain. However, the moment attention is focused on some part of the sensory input, its ascent to perceptual levels is facilitated and there is even some evidence to suggest that emotional states can augment its perceptual impact. The studies of habituation also indicate that the power of a brain to police its own sensory input is no simple matter of closing certain gates and leaving others open according to what the individual has learned from past experience. Instead, it is a dynamic process that is constantly being tuned to the needs of the individual from moment to moment, as his appetites and purposes alter the focus of his attention.

24

Appetitive Sytems in the Brain

I n 1954 I made a trip east to visit a few research laboratories where work of interest to our home team was in progress. One of my ports of call was New Haven, where I visited José Delgado, who told me that he had recently found three pain centers in the monkey brain. By exploring with a needle electrode he had discovered three locations in which an electrical stimulus elicited a behavioral response similar to that which the monkey displayed when a strong electric shock was administered to its feet. José told me that two of these pain centers appeared to be in the hippocampal region, although the exact site of stimulation had not yet been confirmed by microscopic examinations of the brain sections taken from this experimental animal. However, the third site had been confirmed microscopically as being in the midbrain reticular formation at the margin of the central gray matter on its anterolateral aspect. He showed me moving pictures that had been taken of this monkey while this particular midbrain area was being stimulated. These pictures left no doubt that the animal's behavioral response coincided with the onset of the brain stimulation, and the monkey's facial expression and violent struggling certainly suggested that the stimulation was causing pain. I asked to see the microscopic sections showing the exact spot that had been stimulated.

I wanted to see for myself how close this spot was to the area in the cat's midbrain in which we had been able to record responses to tooth-pulp stimuli as they ascended to higher centers in the brain. Although our investigations had been confined to cats and our findings might not be applicable to monkeys, we did not believe that this particular area represented a pain "center." Instead, our observations had indicated that this area was but one of five morphologically distinct "tracts" by which responses to noxious stimuli could ascend the midbrain. Sure enough, an examination of the brain sections of the monkey showed that the tip of the stimulating electrode had been exactly in the area which, in the cat, represented one part of a conducting "system" for pain rather than a true "center" for pain perception. Of course, we could not be sure that this inference drawn from our cat studies would also apply to the monkey, yet both José and I were pleased to find how well our observations had jibed in indicating a direct involvement of the reticular formation in the mechanisms subserving pain perception.

During this same trip I visited Donald Hebb's psychology laboratory at McGill University in Montreal. There I was introduced to a number of young psychologists who were doing interesting studies of rat behavior. Among them were Olds and Milner, who immediately asked me if I would like to see a rat getting "Kickapoo Joy Juice." I had no notion what this meant but said I would be glad to see the rat's response to this juice. They showed me a narrow box in which a white rat, with a needle electrode implanted in its head, was busily pressing on a lever at one end of the box. There was food nearby and plenty of room for the rat to lie down and rest but it apparently was more interested in the lever pressing than anything else. I was told that the tip of the stimulating electrode was in the rat's "septal area" and that each time the lever was depressed an electric shock was administered to the septal region of the rat's brain.

To start this experiment Olds and Milner had found that as soon as the rat had experienced the subjective effects of this electrical stimulation and associated these effects with the lever, it would self-stimulate by the hour. That these subjective experiences were "pleasurable" could be readily demonstrated by interrupting the electrical circuit. The rat soon stopped pressing the lever and turned to the food or lay down to rest, but returned to the lever from time to time to give it a tentative push. If the circuit was still disconnected the rat would depress the lever a time or two and then turn again to the food or lie down. But as soon as the circuit was again activated and the rat discovered this by making a casual push on the lever, it immediately resumed its rapid and persistent self-stimulation (Olds and Milner 1954).

I asked Olds and Milner how they interpreted this remarkable performance. They said they believed that they had discovered a "plea-sure center" in the rat's brain. The reason they thought this area repre-sented a true "center" for pleasure was that they had repeated the same experiment with the electrode in a few other locations without induc-ing the self-stimulation behavior. In fact, when the needle was in the region of the "pain and temperature" tract, the electrical shock seemed to elicit pain in that the rat would immediately squeak and retreat to one corner of the box where it would cower as if trying to get as far away from the lever as possible. In contrast, stimulation in the septal area immediately induced the self-stimulation behavior and the rats "seemed to love it." Olds and Milner felt that the discovery of a true center for pleasure had important philosophical implications. They re-minded me that, whereas the early Greek philosophers had maintained that "pain and pleasure" were the two great motivating forces acting as determinants of behavior, certain modern philosophers were inclined to think that perhaps pain was the only true "drive" and that what the ancients had called pleasure might be merely the "absence of" or the "relief from" pain. But if, as this experiment seemed to demonstrate, the animal brain contains a special center for pleasure, this philosoph-ical problem would be settled in favor of the Greek philosophers.

Subsequent studies by Olds and Milner soon revealed other areas in the rat brain in which electric shocks elicited self-stimulation behavior. It soon was clear that there was no single center for pleasure. Rather, there was an extensive system of neural circuits deep in the basic parts of the brain which, when electrically activated, produced subjective effects that the animal interpreted as rewarding. In fact, activation of portions of this system seemed more rewarding than did food or any other rewards that investigators had been using to induce behavioral responses in experimental animals. Given that no one could know what "feelings" the animal experienced during the stimulation, it was deemed advisable to drop the designation "pleasure" in relation to this system and to say simply that its activation induced "approach" behav-ior. Later, extensive studies of this system by Olds showed that parts were related to the rat's sexual activity because the rate of self-stimula-tion could be modified by castration and the administration of sex hormones. Other parts were definitely related to food or water intake. For example, Olds found two areas in the rat's hypothalamus, very close to each other, both inducing self-stimulation, both related to food intake, and yet having different characteristics. Stimulation of the lateral area increased the rat's appetite for food, while stimulation of the more medial area seemed to induce a feeling of satiety and an avoidance of food (Olds and Olds 1963).

Opposite effects were produced by destructive lesions in these two areas, so that a rat with a laterally placed lesion would starve to death in the presence of food, while a rat with a medially placed lesion might eat so voraciously and continuously that it would become too obese to move. Olds demonstrated another example of the complexity of the "approach" system in the rat. With the stimulating electrode in a particular part of the system, the rat would run across a charged electric grid to press a lever that would start a train of stimuli to its brain and then, as if a point of satiety had been reached, the rat would run back across the grip to press another lever that terminated the train of shocks.

In the meantime, Delgado had been following up his discovery of what he had originally thought were pain centers in the monkey brain (Delgado et al. 1954). He was able to show that there was no true center for pain but rather an extensive system of neural circuits in the brain which, when activated, produced aversive behavior. This system was similar in extent to the approach system and in some areas the two systems were within 2–3 mm of each other. Stimulation of different parts of the aversive system led to different types of behavioral responses in cats and monkeys, but in each instance the behavior clearly indicated that the animal did not like the effects. Both the cats and the monkeys quickly learned to press levers, rotate wheels, or perform other tasks as soon as they discovered that such actions would terminate or prevent electrical shocks delivered to some part of this system.

John Lilly used the monkey's selective response to activation of the two systems to explore their extent (Lilly 1958). For example, he would train a monkey to press a lever to terminate a train of shocks to some part of the aversive system and would permit the monkey to self-stimulate when the electrode was in some part of the approach system. Once so trained, this animal's brain could be explored millimeter by millimeter to map the extent of the two systems. John had used monkeys so often in his experiments and was so familiar with their behavior and dispositions that he felt sure that when a monkey self-stimulated his brain it was because the animal liked the subjective effects. When a part of the aversive system was stimulated, the monkey's behavior seemed to indicate unmistakable "dislike" of the effects. So he preferred to call one system the "I like" system and the other one the "I dislike" system. In his explorations of the "I dislike" system he observed that the monkey's behavior was quite different when the upper and lower limits of this system were activated. When the exploring needle was in this system at the midbrain level a brief electrical stimulation elicited a response that John was sure indicated that the subjective effect was pain. However, when the same stimulus was applied to some part of this system at higher brain levels the monkey's behavior was interpreted as evidence of great fear or "horror."

I visited John's laboratory while his mapping explorations were in progress and I saw for myself these different types of behavioral response when the upper and lower limits of the "I dislike" system were being stimulated in "Pedro," the youngest of his experimental monkeys. Before stimulating Pedro's brain at the lower level of the system, John held a steel rod near Pedro's face, but the monkey just turned his head aside. If it had been a finger Pedro would probably have bitten it but he knew better than to bite a steel rod. Yet, during the brief shock he did bite the rod, broke one of his baby teeth, and reacted as if in a frenzy of pain. His behavior left no doubt in my mind that the experience had been painful to Pedro because it was exactly like the behavioral response of a monkey when powerful electrical shocks are delivered to its feet. But his behavior was quite different when a shock was being delivered to the same system at a higher brain level. Pedro's expression changed the instant the train of stimuli began. His pupils dilated, his hair erected, his mouth formed an "O," and instead of looking at John and me as he had been doing previously, he seemed to be looking beyond us at something that horrified him.

One reason why investigators know so much more about the approach system than they do about the aversive system is that no one likes to cause experimental animals distress of any kind. There can be no doubt that electrical activation of the aversive system is distressing to the animal whether its subjective experiences represent pain or fear, so that these areas are avoided as much as possible in all brain explorations. Nor is the stimulation of such areas entirely free from risk of making the animal seriously ill. Sometimes, after a single stimulation of a particular locus the monkey's appearance and behavior suddenly change; it becomes pale and listless; it is no longer playful or friendly toward its keepers; it loses all interest in food; and it may die unless something is done to restore it. John Lilly has found that the best way to revive such an animal is to permit it to self-stimulate some part of its "I like" system. As the monkey does so, its normal color and activity are quickly restored, it again becomes friendly with its keepers, and its appetite returns to normal. The change in its behavior is just as dramatic as that described in human patients who were permitted to self-stimulate certain parts of their brains, as described in Chapter 19 dealing with the functions of the reticular formation.

As I followed the many investigations of these two great systems I was repeatedly reminded of Aristotle's dissertations on "pleasure and pain." Instead of treating either one as special senses of the body, he dealt with both as inborn "appetites"—one impelling the animal to move toward objects that could satisfy its desires and needs, the other impelling the animal away from objects that might do it harm. Let me quote again one of his statements: "If any order of living things has the sensory, it must also have the appetitive, for appetite is only the genus of which desire, passion and wish are the species; now all animals have one sense at least, viz. touch, and whatever has a sense has the capacity for pleasure and pain, and therefore, has pleasant and painful objects present to it, and wherever these are present, there is desire, for desire is just appetition of what is pleasant."

I like this concept of appetites, with pleasure and pain as the motivating attributes. I prefer to think of these two great natural systems as being appetitive rather than as aversive-approach or "like-dislike" systems. Nor do I think calling one "rewarding" and the other "punishing" quite fills the bill because the cessation of pain often is interpreted as "rewarding" and the long overly stimulation of a reward system may become punishing. The best example of this reversal of "desire" during activation of a single system is the case of the rat that would cross an electrified grid for the privilege of starting a train of stimuli to its brain and then would cross the same grid to terminate the stimulation. We explain such behavior by assuming that a point of "satiety" has been reached, and satiety is the characteristic of all appetites. Every normal human being has experienced satiety as bodily needs change in relation to food, water, sex, and sleep. We are made aware of these changes by an altered "desire" and we are most apt to notice them when they occur within a short period and without "volition." It is easy to think of common examples of such appetitive shifts; how good the sight and smell of food seem when we are hungry and how we resent even the mention of more food when we are stuffed full; how wonderfully good plain water tastes when we have suffered from water depletion; how women seem to acquire a special "aura" to a man after a long period of sexual deprivation; how a placid Siamese cat suddenly turns into a raving maniac when she is in heat; how pleasant it is, after climbing a mountain all day, to lie down on the rocks and go to sleep under conditions that would be intolerable in any other body state.

These are a few of the reasons why I like to think of activity in these newly discovered systems as appetites that are constantly fluctuating in terms of bodily needs. What we call them isn't as important as simply knowing that they exist. I find it exciting to know that they are there in the brain of a newborn infant because it seems to me that they provide the final ingredient necessary for the creation of a mind. The other ingredients are already there: a sensory system to bring in information from the external and internal environments, a motor system to respond to this input, and an interposed brain component with the capacity to store information and use it again in fashioning the appropriate motor response. These three systems provide the ingredients necessary for "learning," while the appetitive systems add the *incentives* for learning. The baby's behavior reflects the state of activity in these systems from the moment of birth. Without volition or anything that might be called thinking, the baby feels drawn toward objects and people that promise comfort and drawn away from those that cause it distress. Long before the growing infant can express its preferences by movements toward or away from external objects, its behavior clearly reflects its subjective feelings of pleasure or distress. The "traces" left in its brain nets by the reiterated sensory impressions coming in from the outside world eventually lead the child to associate objects and people with the affective states they elicit. These associations in turn eventually lead to recognition of certain people and things and to increasingly selective behaviors in relation to them. I believe that it is at this point, when the baby begins to make discriminative choices, that its mind is born. From this point on, its choices become increasingly discriminative and its efforts to move toward sources of pleasure and away from sources of discomfort, fear, and pain become increasingly effective. Now, truly, we can say that the baby has a mind of its own.

In closing this chapter I might add one more speculative excursion in this discussion of the two great appetitive systems. I have been impressed by the observations of many investigators who suggest that electrical stimulation of the posterior portion of the "I dislike" system causes pain, while the same stimulation to the system at higher levels elicits responses suggestive of fear or horror. Stimulation of other portions of the system may elicit subjective sensations that are harder to classify but that are always distressing. Sem-Jacobsen (1968) has apparently activated such intermediate areas in human patients. They are unable to describe the sensations the stimulus elicits. When they try to describe what they felt, words seem to fail them beyond saying that the sensory experience was unlike any sensation they had ever known previously, that it was "awful," and please don't stimulate that spot again. Observations of this kind remind me that I have almost as much difficulty in defining such words as fear or pain in terms of a single specific sensation as I would in trying to define "awful" in similar terms. My point is that I am beginning to wonder if the gamut of sensory experiences we are accustomed to calling pain might be due to the activation of some part of the "I dislike" system. I am also beginning to wonder if the best way to control pain might not be to activate some portion of the "I like" system. I do not mean that I think everyone should be provided with a button to press to relieve pain by brain stimulation, as Robert Heath has done with some of his patients and was done recently at the Massachusetts General Hospital to relieve the intolerable pain of a man dying of inoperable cancer of the pharynx. I would hope that simpler means might be found to accomplish this purpose. It is certainly worth shooting for.

25

Pulling the Picture Together

In dealing with so many different subjects that have no obvious connection, it might appear that I had forgotten the evolving ideal that was supposed to be the central theme of this narrative. On the contrary, it has been there in the background all the time, serving to hold these subjects in context and evolving under their influence. Now I feel obligated to haul it back into the foreground to see what has been happening to it and what future changes might be anticipated. For the time has come, as artists say, to "try to pull the picture together." This is sound advice for would-be painters and narrators alike but it can have a paralyzing effect on an amateur who has no notion of how to go about it. That is my predicament. I am oppressed by all the questions I am unable to answer, reluctant to reveal my uncertainties, and unable to decide how to wind up a story that is so far from finished. I am sorely tempted to stop right here. I might excuse the abrupt ending by saying that I wanted the reader to be entirely free to accept or reject whatever parts of the story he wishes in the formulation or reevaluation of his own concept of pain. But this would be merely an excuse and an evasion of the responsibility I voluntarily assumed when I offered to give a frank account of all that seems to me to have happened to my concept of pain during my professional lifetime. I suppose some recapitulation is in order, but how shall I begin? Well, if I want to avoid one of the criticisms Polybius (c205–c123 B.C.E.) aimed at the chronicles of his contemporary Greek historians, I ought to "refer to the starting point and show how and why that point led to the transactions of the moment."

The personalized part of my story started with the "opening of a colostomy." I had been informed that there is only one specific pain fiber, but I was forced to wonder if there might not be at least two. I wondered, too, if pain was really measurable in terms of stimulus intensity or the force of the reflex responses to the injury inflicted by the noxious stimulus. In my search for an answer to what I thought was a simple question about visceral sensibility, I got little help from physiologists. On the other hand, I discovered that many very wise clinicians had thought about it much more deeply than I and had linked it with the problem of "referred phenomena." The three men who seemed to have thought most deeply about this obscure problem all seemed to feel that pain was not always a simple "from-here-to-there" problem of direct transmission, but probably involved some change of function within the central nervous system. Later, I made observations indicating that visceral afferents might change their unresponsiveness to many stimuli and that in the presence of chronic inflammation or other forms of prolonged irritation might even respond to "touch." For example, one of my friends who specialized in gastrointestinal disturbances told me jokingly that some of his patients with ulcerative colitis could "tell when a kernel of hominy passed their splenic flexure."

As my clinical practice increased, I began to encounter chronic pain states, major and minor causalgias, phantom limb pains, glomus tumors, "mirror images," and other bizarre manifestations of pain that suggested that the central nervous system was playing an active part in sustaining, if not in creating, chronic pain states. More and more my push-button concept of pain seemed to be changing under the influence of clinical observations. But a clinician's speculations about what such observations might mean must have support from specialists in other lines of inquiry before they mean much.

In 1947 I joined a team of investigators willing to combine forces in a study of pain phenomena. We were held together by the common desire to learn more about human pain problems. We felt that to do this demanded a knowledge of the perceptual aspects of pain and information about its possible neural substrates. Our ultimate aim was to establish some correlation between these two important aspects of pain. We also agreed that what was most important to the patient was the severity of the pain he felt as opposed to what we thought he ought to be feeling or even what nerve impulses might be ascending his central

The discovery that had the most direct
bearing on our pain problem
was that the brain possesses the power
to modulate its own sensory input
and it may exert this influence
all the way out to the sensory
receptor ending.

nervous system when his tissues were being cut by the surgeon's knife while he was deeply anesthestized. So we subscribed to the proposition that *nothing can properly be called "pain" unless it can be consciously perceived as such.* In the course of our laboratory investigations we discovered that responses to tooth-pulp stimulation in cats ascended the classical "pain pathway" best when the brain was deeply anesthetized. In contrast, in the alert state these responses followed other routes up the core of the brain. It further seemed that these newly discovered routes had more to do with pain "perception" than did the classical route. These core routes proved to be highly susceptible to temporarily acting analgesics, such as nitrous oxide and intravenous procaine, and we were able to use this fact as an exploratory tool in our studies.

In the meantime, a revolution was occurring in neurophysiology that made it necessary for us to reorganize or abandon many of our basic concepts of function. The discovery that had the most direct bearing on our pain problem was that the brain possesses the power to modulate its own sensory input and it may exert this influence all the way out to the sensory receptor ending. The important thing about this discovery was that this ability to suppress incoming patterns was exerted at levels far below any possible perceptual level. If this were true, we must question the assumption made according to the push-button concept that pain was always directly proportional to stimulus intensity. We even began to wonder if, when our attention was diverted from some chronic pain, it might not only *seem* less but actually *be* less. All this made us doubt the validity of our attempt to draw a clear distinction between a patient's pain and his reaction to it.

As the effects of the "interpretive" revolution changed our concept of central nervous system function, the mechanistic shortcomings of the push-button concept became increasingly evident. Nevertheless, we continued to use it in our daily conversations and even relied on parts of it in some of our investigations and interpretations. For example, when Hagbarth and Kerr (1954) demonstrated to us that intercurrent stimulation of certain parts of the brain cut in half the amplitude of responses ascending the pain and temperature tract, we accepted this demonstration as an indication that the brain has the power to inhibit pain. We didn't always stop to distinguish between a signal that might subserve pain and pain itself, unless we wanted to be exact in our language. Common sense told us that human beings must have sensory systems that usually bring them reliable reports of what is happening peripherally and all these systems must behave much alike, otherwise we would not all use the same terms for noxious stimulation such as pricking, cutting, burning, aching, cramping, etc.—words that a physician finds so useful in helping to recognize the nature and possible source of a patient's hidden pain. The push-button concept was in common use and as long as we understood its limitations, we would continue to use it or at least parts of it. But our laboratory studies and our experience in treating chronic pain states have also convinced us that the push-button concept is only one part of a much more complex entity and is of no real use to us in accounting for what might be called "pathological pain." Without intending to make any odious comparisons, I might say that our attitude toward the push-button concept is much like the attitude we might assume had we been listening to one of the blind men describe an elephant after he had palpated only that animal's trunk. We might praise him for giving such a clever account of the most characteristic and useful parts of an elephant, and yet we would still have to say that he wasn't describing a living elephant.

In view of these considerations I will defer my attempt to describe my present concept of pain to a final chapter entitled "Interpretations and Speculations." First, it seems advisable to examine the main postulates of the push-button concept to see what parts might be useful to retain and what parts should be discarded. It should be clear that I am approaching it in a friendly fashion, but also equally clear that the examination should be critical, even fussy, in order to eliminate any parts that might restrict our understanding of human pain problems.

The Punctate Theory and the Specific Pain Fiber

The original assumption that pressure on a "skin spot" activates only one specifically adapted sensory fiber is no longer tenable. Everyone now concedes that pressure with von Frey hairs and most other forms of skin stimulation must activate many sensory fibers of different sizes and conduction rates. However, there is good evidence to show that sensory fibers in the skin are often highly selective in their ability to respond to particular types of skin stimulation. Tasaki has recorded responses to stimulation in individual sensory fibers supplied to the skin and has classified them into touch, pressure, nociceptive, cold, wide-receptive, hair, scratch, and unmyelinated mechanoreceptors.[1] He gives them these names to indicate the particular types of stimulation needed to activate each kind. He used these descriptive words because he knew that physiologists would understand that he was referring to *physiological* specificity in the fibers themselves. But Tasaki was not pretending to say what sensory experiences the cat might be having during his tests, had the cat been awake and capable of describing its subjective experiences. Physiological specificity can be defined in terms of "stimulus," that is, the fiber's selective response to particular chemical and physical perturbations, but this kind of specificity cannot be identified by such words as touch, pain, heat, and cold, as these words have been used in the past to describe specific sensory experiences. Certainly I have found nothing in Tasaki's observations to suggest that he thinks any one of the fibers he tested in a cat subserves pain and no other sensation.

Furthermore, these four words denote sensory experiences that have no fixed connotation and are relative to many factors, both external and internal to the perceiving individual. Tepid water feels cool to

---

[1]*Editor's Note:* I have not been able to find work by Tasaki on this subject. The earliest published accounts of single-fiber recordings of nociceptors that would have been available to Livingston would have been by Iggo in 1959 and 1960; Iriuchijima and Zotterman 1960, and Witt 1962. For reviews of this early literature see Chapters 2 (by Burgess and Perl) and 3 (by Hensel) in *Somatosensory System. Handbook of Sensory Physiology,* Vol. II, A Iggo (Ed). Berlin: Springer-Verlag, 1973, pp 29–110.

our skin after long immersion in hot water, but the same water feels warm to us after long exposure to cold. A skin contact that would be described as touch to normal skin would be called pain if applied to sunburned skin and might be intolerably painful when applied to the affected extremity of a person suffering from major causalgia.

When the push-button concept was formulated it was assumed that all different kinds of pain were subserved by a single, specifically adapted pain fiber. Now we talk about "slow" pain and "fast" pain and ascribe the slow kind to very tiny, nonmedullated fibers of the C group and the fast kind to small myelinated fibers of the A group, in the gamma-delta elevation. The only morphological feature these two widely different sensory fibers have in common is that their endings are undifferentiated, the kind we call "naked" terminals. The sensory fibers supplied to the cornea of the eye all have naked endings and as long as this delicate structure was assumed to have only pain sensibility, it did not seem unreasonable to assume that they represented specific pain fibers. But this argument has lost its force with the demonstration that the cornea also possesses touch and temperature sensibility.

Finally, there is little doubt that all sensory experiences we derive from skin stimulation are much more complex than they seem in that the sensory nerves are constantly bringing us a great deal more information than we can interpret. The situation is illustrated by our ability to distinguish the sounds of particular musical instruments. If we hear an instrument sound a tone, we usually can identify the instrument producing it according to what we hear. We know that its characteristic tone is due to the relationships between the various overtones it produces and we realize that our ability to name the instrument means that we must be hearing a highly complex combination of sounds, yet few people are able to identify them. The same thing could be said about all our sensory systems, that they can provide us with a wealth of information if only we took the trouble to "read" it discriminatively as do the wine-tasters, "trackers," and the gifted musicians who "hear" a new score as they look at it. As I think about these sensory resources most of us leave untapped, three pictures come vividly to my mind: I "see" Helen Keller delicately palpating Eleanor Roosevelt's face; Major Jim Corbett moving quietly through the jungle, all his senses so alert that they almost suggest delicate antennae all tuned to "tiger"; and the amazement on the faces of my colleagues the first time we both saw and heard recordings taken from the midbrain reticular formation of an unanesthetized brain. In view of all this, such words as touch, pain, heat, and cold seem to lose all claim to represent "primary" sensations, and the effort to identify each one with a single neural unit strikes me as almost childish. In the next section of this chapter I will set forth and critically examine some commonly held but, I believe, incomplete assumptions that limit our ability to understand the nature of pain.

Assumption 1. The anterolateral spinothalamic tract is "the pain and temperature tract."

The idea that the anterolateral spinothalamic tract is the pain and temperature tract is unquestionably the most reliable part of the push-button concept. No one can challenge the fact that when sensory impulse patterns enter the spinal cord they are sorted out in some mysterious fashion so that most of those subserving pain and temperature sensibility enter this particular specialized and fast-conducting fiber tract, while most of those subserving proprioceptive and touch sensibility ascend in other equally specialized tracts. The easiest way to account for this fact would be to assume, as we did in the past, that pain must reach the spinal cord in a specific pain fiber that makes direct synaptic connection with the secondary neuron whose fiber ascends to the thalamus in the pain and temperature tract. In fact, this interpretation has long been used as the mainstay of the push-button concept; one is almost tempted to call it the "backbone" of the concept. However, as we learn more about the dynamic activity within the "internuncial pools" through which the sensory input must pass, the downstream influences exerted on it by way of the reticular formation, and the transactional nature of all neural functioning, we must conclude that the idea of pattern is superseding the idea of direct transmission of unprocessed pain signal. The notion that the very existence of a pain and temperature tract is proof of the specificity of pain seems to be fading. It was once argued that pain has already been tied into a neat package in the spinal cord so that it could be delivered rapidly and directly to a special pain center in the brain. Such packages may serve as useful conceptual devices in teaching medical students, but they often come "untied" again at higher levels. This is what seems to happen in the case of the pain and temperature tract. In the midbrain it is seen to peter out and the information it had carried up the cord so compactly is delivered to many parts of the brain other than the cerebral cortex.

There is no need to prolong this discussion by considering all the pros and cons of cordotomy. I would not deny the possible benefit of this operation to some poor devil in the terminal stages of cancer if I could not control his pain in any other way. But I am certainly not enthusiastic about the procedure, perhaps because the chronic pain states that present my most serious clinical problems seem to be the ones least likely to be relieved by a cordotomy. I am glad that this operation has been added to our armamentarium for fighting pain but I would be inclined to use it as the last shot in the locker. Both clinical and experimental evidence confirm that pain "signals" can reach perceptual levels by other, less direct routes in the spinal cord and brainstem.

Assumption 2. **The sensory area of the cerebral cortex is the center for pain perception.**

Enough has been said about this assumption to make it unnecessary to reemphasize the importance of subcortical structures in all perceptual processes. However, this does not rule out an important role for the cerebral cortex in pain perception. Responses to all forms of noxious stimulation occur in somatosensory cortex and they must participate in some way in pain perception even though their amplitude is greatest and they are most easily recorded when the brain is anesthetized. The somatosensory cortex area provides a more accurate topographical map of the body as it exists in space than do any of the subcortical structures, so it can be assumed that the cortex aids in the localization of a noxious stimulus and probably plays a part in our ability to discriminate between the many different kinds of pain. But we know nothing about how this process contributes to a pain perception.

Assumption 3. **Pain is measurable in terms of stimulus intensity.**

It would be of enormous value to the clinician have a testing device that would accurately indicate on its dial the intensity of a patient's pain. Earnest efforts have been made to devise some instrument or method to measure pain objectively. I have participated in this search and have tested on myself several devices that were claimed to measure pain according to some definite scale of values. Fred Haugen and I conducted a study of the "dolorimeter" as a measuring device and performed innumerable tests on each other over two years in an attempt to evaluate the usefulness of a "dol scale." We still carry scars from deep burns acquired in testing what has been called the ultimate ceiling for pain, but we were never able to convince ourselves, as some have claimed, that the pain one suffers from a locally destructive burn of this kind was as great as if one were being burned at the stake. Our observations have been reported elsewhere together with our conclusion that the dolorimeter may have some limited usefulness in testing

---

We still carry scars from deep burns acquired in testing what has been called the ultimate ceiling for pain, but we were never able to convince ourselves, as some have claimed, that the pain one suffers from a locally destructive burn of this kind was as great as if one were being burned at the stake.

---

pain in an experimental laboratory but it can contribute little of value to the study of chronic pain states. At one stage in our study of this instrument we were cocky enough to think we could guess the intensity of the heat stimulus in the number of dols we were experiencing. I can vouch for the fact that when every condition was "just right" in the isolated room in which our tests were conducted and I could give my full attention to the test, there was a reasonable correlation between the instrumental readings and the intensity of the pain I experienced. But if my skin was beginning to get the least bit irritated by successive tests, if I was startled by a rapid increase of the heat that threatened a burn, or if anything happened to divert my attention from the test, my judgments went completely haywire.

Some of the factors that can affect tests of this kind can be illustrated by an amusing story told me by Joe Hinsey. In Joe's laboratory, researchers were using a dolorimeter to stimulate the back of a man's hand to determine whether the vasomotor responses to the pain stimulus, as recorded from the fingers of the stimulated hand, differed in time of onset or degree from any vasomotor changes that could be recorded from the fingers of the opposite hand. The heat from the dolorimeter was adjusted so that the test subject's "pain threshold" would be reached within the three seconds that the dolorimeter shutter remained open. One finger of each hand was encased in an "oncometer" (a device to measure volume changes), the subject was blindfolded, and the changes in finger volume in the two fingers were visualized and recorded. At the instant the subject's pain threshold was reached, a quick change in blood volume (vasoconstriction) occurred in the fingers of both hands that was both simultaneous and equal in degree, although only one hand was receiving the pain stimulus. The experimenter was using a telegraph key to open the dolorimeter shutter and the closing of this key made a faint click. But it happened that occasionally the shutter stuck and the hand did not get the usual pain stimulus. However, even in the absence of the pain stimulus, the same sudden shift in blood volume occurred exactly as it would be expected to do had the pain stimulus been given. This response in the absence of a painful stimulus was obviously a conditioned response. The blindfolded subject evidently had learned to associate the faint click with the anticipated pain stimulus, so that this sound alone was enough to initiate the vasomotor response, exactly as the ringing of a bell could start salivation in one of Pavlov's conditioned dogs.

The psychologist expressed an interest in seeing the dolorimeter and offered to serve as a test subject himself. When he came to the laboratory for this purpose, he was blindfolded and the oncometers were put on his two index fingers. As this was being done the experimenter cautioned the psychologist against moving during the test by saying that even the slightest movement of the fingers would spoil the recordings. The explanation for this caution went something like this: "Professor, when the shutter opens you will feel an increasing sensation of heat. This feeling will build up so fast that you may be tempted to jerk your hand away for fear of being burned." At the mention of the word "burned" a beautiful recording was made of the typical vasomotor change in his fingers—no burning and no conditioning, just a suggestion.

One further comment might be added about all attempts to measure pain objectively. Their primary purpose, as I understand it, is to help a clinician evaluate the patient's complaints of pain in terms of his "physical pain" and his "reaction" to it. The implication is that the physical pain is a constant in terms of stimulus strength, and though it inevitably registers in consciousness, the individual can elect to disregard it—or his fears and other emotions can make it *seem* worse than it actually is. There is little doubt that our attitude toward a pain has a great deal to do with our ability to tolerate it. Every experienced clinician has had patients coming to him complaining of severe pain that they fear is the first sign of cancer, and has seen that pain reduced to negligible proportions an soon as the patient's fears have been allayed. Knowing these things, I can appreciate the value of making a clear distinction between physical pain and reaction to it, so that each factor can be given appropriate treatment. But for myself, the more I have studied a wide variety of causalgic states and even the ordinary, persistent pain of patients, the less confident I am of my ability to clearly establish this line of demarcation. And, as I have said previously, now that I know that the patient's own central nervous system possesses the power to influence its sensory input before he can perceive it, I am still less confident of my ability to make such judgments and am increasingly reluctant to hang on my patient such labels as psychasthenia, hysteria, and malingering.

Finally, since the discovery of the two appetitive systems in the brain, one at the midbrain level that responds to direct electrical stimulation with every manifestation of severe pain and other at some higher level that responds with behavior more suggestive of fear and horror, I am beginning to wonder if our whole concept of pain may not need a careful review. And, though I dread it, this is what I shall try to do as frankly as I know how and from my own point of view in the closing chapter.

26

Interpretations and Speculations

I n this final countdown, I am supposed to bring my story of an evolving idea up to date. To pick up the idea where we last left it, we must turn back to determine its status as depicted in *Pain Mechanisms* more than twenty years ago. There were two reasons why I felt impelled to write this book. The first was that the orthodox teachings about pain failed to account for the most serious pain problems a clinician must deal with, in which the pain did not seem to arise at the periphery but from irritation of nerve trunks, roots, and spinal cord and which could lead to disturbances of function within the central nervous system itself. The second reason was that I hoped the implications of the internuncial pool concept might assist in ridding orthodox teachings about sensory physiology from their tendency to identify a "sensation" with a particular form of stimulation and to use oversimplified diagrams and mechanistic interpretations. Here is an example of what I mean, taken from a relatively recent "review": "Knowledge concerning the primary sensory systems is well established and a part of neurological orthodoxy. Each of these systems, from specific receptor through laterally situated lemniscal pathways to localized cortical zone, is sensitive to a single modality of sensation."

In Chapter 12 I described some of the clinical interpretations recorded in *Pain Mechanisms*, but in this chapter I wish only to record my groping efforts to express my own concept of pain as a "perceptual process." Here are the propositions.

1. Pain is a perception and as such is subject to the influence of associated ideas, apperceptions, and fears.

217

2. The impulses that subserve it are not pain but are merely a part of its underlying and alterable mechanisms.

3. The impulses may be initiated by a wide variety of stimuli; they are probably picked up by more than one type of receptor end-organ; certainly they are carried by fibers of widely variant diameters and at quite different velocities.

4. When they enter the spinal cord they are subject to modification by the internuncial pool of central neurons, whose activity is determined from moment to moment by other sensory impulses and by influences from other parts of the central nervous system.

5. In their ascent to higher centers the impulses are subject to further modification at each functional level, the modifications at the various levels constituting an integration that strongly influences the sensation ultimately perceived.

6. In the sensorium they register as a pattern of excitation and from the resultant complex of sensory impressions, particular sensations such as pain may be recognized as the dominant feature.

These propositions were admittedly speculative and reported as impressions when I published my book on pain mechanisms (Livingston 1943) twenty years ago. However, in the final chapter of that book I ventured these additional comments:

> On a few points only, I have what might be called convictions. I believe that the concept of 'specificity' when used to identify sensory experiences with particular end-organs and nerve fibers has led away from a true perspective. I am convinced that it is a mistake to assume that a certain pain syndrome must represent an 'obsession,' or be of purely 'psychic' origin, simply because its manifestations do not conform to what we have been taught about the anatomy and physiology of peripheral nerve pathways. I believe that it is equally foolish to discredit the results of procedures, such as a periarterial sympathectomy and novocaine injection, on the ground that their mode of action is obscure. I am convinced that the whole story of causalgia will not be learned from a study of the functions of the sympathetic nerves. Beyond these few convictions, my impressions are still too plastic to be called conclusions.

Four years after *Pain Mechanisms* was published, I joined the team of investigators the University of Oregon Medical School. During the eleven years we worked together my concept of pain was profoundly influenced by the investigations and wise counsel of my colleagues. We agreed that *no* mechanistic concept of pain, certainly not one based on the study of "normal" test subjects, could be used to account for the human pain problems we encountered in our clinics. We found entirely unconvincing the evidence offered in support of the notion that pain was the direct result of activation of specific sensory receptors at the body periphery. The most characteristic feature of the cases we studied was a profound disturbance of normal sensibility at the periphery and its cause seemed to be higher up along conducting pathways or within the central nervous system. We had ample evidence that the pain and temperature tract in the spinal cord was not the sole route by which pain signals could ascend to perceptual levels, because signals could take many indirect routes and back doors to bypass any point of interruption of this tract. Finally, our laboratory studies indicated that the cerebral cortex was not the true center for pain perception, as responses to noxious stimuli could take other routes in the core of the brain to reach subcortical structures and areas of the cortex outside the somatosensory region.

In the meantime, studies in other laboratories revealed the enormous importance of the "transactional" component of the brain and showed that the all-or-none principle applied only to the axon of the single neuron. The finding of stretch receptors and gamma efferents was complicating our concept of the reflex. We learned that the brain exerts a "downstream" influence on all sensory input. Animal studies demonstrated that behavior could be controlled through two appetitive systems.

The effect was to make our concept of pain more complex and more dynamic and thus harder to express concisely, but at the same time, these findings held out hope that neural correlates might eventually be established that could explain a broader range of pain perceptions. We felt that our original decision had been vindicated, i.e., that "nothing can properly be called 'pain' unless it can be consciously perceived as such." It no longer seemed necessary to deal with pain as a "sensation" devoid of perceptual aspects. Indeed, the obnoxious qualities of all pains *demand* attention and action! The person may elect to ignore a particular pain or may decide that it needs further attention, but in either event, the person must first "perceive" it and reach some decision as to its possible significance. If he fears that it implies some threat to his life or health and he focuses his attention on it, the pain not only seems worse, it is worse! If he decides that it is safe to ignore the pain and turn his attention to other things, the pain not only *seems* less, it *is* less! Finally, our evolving concept of pain suggested new avenues of approach to the treatment of human pain problems, all of which seemed worthy of serious investigation. As this is not a clinical dissertation, I will merely list some of these suggested approaches, with only brief comments.

1. An earnest effort should be made to determine the pain-controlling influence of various forms of conditioning, progressive relaxation training, hypnotism, etc. (Personally, I believe that the conditioning a child receives from parental influences can change the severity of the pains he will experience for the remainder of his life.)

2. If pain can originate from multiple sources that perturb function within the central nervous system and this lowers the person's pain threshold, the sum total of the pain might be whittled down and the threshold raised by removing as many of the accessible sources of irritation as possible. (For example, we have been successful in markedly raising the exercise level of cardiac patients exhibiting the so-called "effort syndrome" by using procaine infiltration to eliminate "trigger points" in the muscles and fascia of their chest and shoulders.)

3. There may be other ways in which a central perturbation of function might be influenced, such as the intravenous injection of dilute solution of procaine solution, prolonged cooling of the body, or protracted periods of sleep. (In our pain clinic we have found that intravenous procaine is often successful in lessening the severity of certain types of chronic pain that we have been unable to relieve in any other way.)

4. Various types of "nerve block" with temporarily acting local anesthetic drugs need further study, although nerve block has already demonstrated its usefulness in controlling pain by its action on nerve trunks, plexuses, bathing the spinal nerve roots, and direct infiltrations of sympathetic ganglia. (We have had success using procaine injections of sympathetic ganglia and different types of sympathectomy and ramicotomy to relieve certain pains involving the extremities, although we know little of their relation to pain pathways.)

Finally, I might add a few comments on future investigations of pain phenomena. We know something about the routes in the midbrain by which responses to tooth-pulp stimulation ascend to higher levels in the brain. We have reason to believe these responses have something to do with pain perception and we have traced some responses bilaterally to the second face area of the cortex. We also know that all these responses except the one in the trigeminal lemniscus are depressed in a characteristic fashion by a few inhalations of ether or nitrous oxide and also by very small intravenous doses of procaine. We had already used this fact to distinguish trigeminal lemniscus responses from spinothalamic responses in the primary face area. All three of these drugs have an analgesic effect in humans, and the changes they elicit in the responses to noxious stimuli in the cat brain suggest that they are also analgesic for lower animals. These observations suggest two possibilities: first, that the midbrain level might be a good place to test the analgesic effects of other drugs; and second, that by carrying these investigations to higher levels we may catch our first glimpse of the neural correlates of a perception. This is all very speculative but it explains why I think that pain may prove a valuable "tool" in exploring the neural basis for perception.[1]

Let me close with a fanciful parable. A philosopher and a physiologist are arguing about pain. The philosopher insists that it is an affective state of the mind, while the physiologist is equally sure that it is a strictly physical sensation. The physiologist wants to keep the argument on a strictly objective scientific basis and, because he believes that words like "mind" tend to foster the old idea of a dichotomy between mind and body, which he considers a misconception, he wants to deal with pain as a sensation devoid of perceptual aspects. The physiologist is apparently unaware that by so doing, he is himself fostering the idea of a dichotomy. Anyway, he insists that pain is a sensation and he first identifies it with a noxious stimulus, then with naked sensory receptor endings, then with a pain fiber, then with a tract in the spinal cord, and then with a particular spot in the cerebral cortex. While he has been making this trip from stimulus to body surface and then up the three units in the pain pathway, a revolution in neurophysiological methods

---

[1]*Editor's Note:* Chapter 26 originally included material related to a set of slides that we did not receive with the manuscript. We have moved text related to the slides and edited the last two paragraphs to improve cohesiveness and flow. The omitted material has been edited and included in Appendix D as some readers will find it interesting or illuminating. It will also allow an assessment of the validity of the edits.

has occurred and through recordings and stimulation of the brain in awake human beings, the physiologist is arriving at not a "mind" but a "mind-brain" that has become accessible to his exploring electrodes.

What I am trying to suggest by this vague parable is that perhaps, as we learn more about the brain mechanisms of what I call the "appetitive" systems, the interpretations of pain by philosophers and physiologists alike may find a common ground of understanding. In these symptoms may lie that "specificity" the physiologist has been searching for, originating in the design of the brain itself and not specific receptors in the periphery or in individual neural units in a conducting pathway. Here may lie the seat of the "affective states" the philosopher has been talking about, not in some ephemeral "mind" that has no neural correlates. From this thought experiment, we might begin to understand the brain as evolving throughout the millenia in a continual pattern of change that best serves the individual's need for protection of self and perpetuation of his species. To do this the individual's nervous system must be patterned for action, provided with a sensory system that maintains contact with the internal and external environments, and equipped with a transactional component that integrates both input and output. Underneath these three must lie a "like-dislike" component that will help guide the individual in making the choices that best serve body needs and the needs of the species. Yet, I cannot see these systems as "yes-no" components of fixed value but rather as flexible systems that are constantly being tuned to the body's needs, desires, and purposes.

Appendices

The publication of *Pain and Suffering* more than thirty years after Livingston's death necessitated editorial revisions to the original manuscript. The twenty-six chapters, written over ten years, were in different stages of development; some were close to final, others were in rough draft. Minor editorial revisions included updating the text to conform to current conventions of grammar, spelling, and style, modifying colloquialisms, and clarifying some statements and deleting others that could not be interpreted. More significant revisions included changing the order of several chapters and moving some material to the appendices to improve the text flow. An appendix referred to in the original text evidently was never completed or was lost. Dr. Ronald Melzack has made an effort to partially reconstruct it as Appendix B.

The manuscript did not include any bibliographic material beyond author names and publication dates cited in the text; consequently, the references in this book are my best guess as to Dr. Livingston's source material. Javid Ghandehari assisted me in bibliographic research. My confidence in the accuracy of individual references ranges from total to slight. In a few instances I was unable to find a useful citation for the material. I accept responsibility for any misinterpretations or mistaken attributions that might have resulted from my editorial and bibliographic work on this book.

HOWARD L. FIELDS, MD, PHD
Editor

Appendix A

Discussion from 1938 Paper

The ten cases of post-traumatic pain syndrome presented in this and the preceding paper have been drawn from a larger series of cases having fundamentally similar characteristics. In introducing these case histories I have already given the essential features of my own interpretation of the phenomena reported, but it seems worthwhile, before elaborating this view, to consider briefly several fundamental questions that any critical consideration of these cases must raise.

First, are these patients psychoneurotics or do they have organic pathology?

It is my opinion that an organic lesion is present in each instance no matter what evidences of "psychoneurosis" may have been present before or after the pain syndrome develops. It is quite possible that certain individuals, or any individual in prepared states of the central nervous system equilibrium, may be more prone to develop intractable pain syndromes than others. But such a statement is purely speculative and even the terminology is too vague to mean much. Certainly, if one admits the organic nature of the original injury and the reality of the symptoms, it might be expected that the irritation to the central nervous system from a continuous assault by pain impulses, could exaggerate any predisposition to "neurotic" signs and symptoms, or actually create them where none existed previously.

I realize that this is a dangerous doctrine. It is particularly dangerous to the industrial surgeon who has to deal with borderline and difficult diagnostic problems in his office and in the courts. I am also aware that there are definite cases of psychoneurosis and malingering

225

which can be proved to be exceptions to the above statements, and that the distinguishing of one type from the others may be most difficult. But my contention is, that as knowledge of the pathological physiology of the central nervous system increases, particularly that related to pain phenomena, diagnosis of "psychoneurosis" and "malingering" will be used with less frequency.

In support of my view I need but mention the excessive pain reactions accompanying a causalgia or an ischemic paralysis. Two factors contribute to prevent patients with either of these syndromes from being classed as malingerers: the obvious trophic changes that take place in the limb and the fact that master surgeons have described them as clinical entities. In the causalgia cases it has come to be recognized that a partial severance of a major nerve is responsible for the condition and that resection of the damaged portion and end-to-end suture of the nerve *may* cure the syndrome or that a sympathectomy may alleviate or abolish it. From a study of causalgia surgeons have come to recognize that an irritative lesion to nerve fibers may be of much more serious consequence to the individual than complete severance of the nerve trunk. In ischemic paralysis no less striking subjective and objective changes occur and yet no one has been able to demonstrate the specific lesion responsible for its production, although the view is commonly expressed that it is dependent upon nerve irritation and nerve reflexes.

I believe that the cases here reported are of close kin to both causalgia and ischemic paralysis. There may be other clinical entities which future investigations will prove to have some relationship. Trigeminal neuralgia, meralgia paresthetica, the cervical rib syndrome, phantom limb pain, and possibly such conditions as angina pectoris, migraine, and some types of neuralgia may be dependent upon nerve reflexes and might conceivably originate from an organic trigger point. Some of the patients in the present series described pain that was very similar to that suffered by patients with trigeminal neuralgia, and it may be significant that an injection of procaine solution has been known abolish the pain attacks in a typical tic douloureux. However, these additional clinical entities are mentioned only as *possibly* having a relationship, whereas the parallelism between my cases and causalgia and ischemic paralysis is so complete as to suggest a common etiology.

Second, can a local injury give rise to profound and diffuse nerve reflexes?

The meticulous investigations by Sir Thomas Lewis and his colleagues into the mechanism causing the hyperalgesia which follows local trauma would answer at least a part of this question in the affirmative. He has shown that following injury to small areas of skin or faradic stimulation of sensory nerves there develops a local tenderness and sometimes an hyperalgesia over a considerable area of skin near the lesion. From well-controlled experiments he deduces that the hyperalgesia develops in the absence of sympathetic or ventral root influences and is dependent upon axon reflexes in neurons having their cell bodies in the posterior root ganglia. He believes that these axon reflex impulses bring about some alteration in the cells of the skin, which causes them to elaborate substances that act locally to reduce the threshold of pain nerves. He further concludes from the widespread effect produced, that the involved nerve fiber must arborize freely in the skin and hence cannot be the ordinary sensory neuron because if such arborizations existed in a single sensory nerve fiber, accurate localization of sensation would not be possible. He therefore postulates the existence of a new system of hitherto unknown neurons which he calls the "nocifensors" because they have to do with defense mechanisms. Whether or not this postulation of a new system of nerves is necessary to explain his experimental evidence is beside the point here. The important point is that in these and other equally brilliant contributions from his laboratory he has established beyond question that minor types of injury can call forth local and even widespread changes in sensation and the activity of the arterioles and capillaries and that these changes are dependent upon nerve reflexes.

That the reflexes which Lewis is investigating are mediated through the posterior root ganglia does not in any way argue that other reflexes over other pathways and perhaps even more widespread in their effects may not take place as a result of injury or nerve irritation.

Third, may the sympathetic nervous system become involved in reflex disturbances originating from a local peripheral injury?

The cases presented in these papers would seem to indicate that it can and does. They would further imply that reflexes acting over the sympathetic nerves can produce very localized as well as generalized effects. The objection might be raised that the sympathetic nervous system is not constructed for segmental and local reflexes. The general concept seems to be that, whereas the parasympathetic system is adapted to specific and localized reflex effects, the sympathetic system is fashioned for the dissemination of impulses over large parts of the body simultaneously. Yet there is evidence to support the view that the sympathetic nerves *can* take part in localized reflex responses. Segmental contraction of arteries following trauma usually occurs in the limb sustaining the injury, but is occasionally expressed in the contralateral limb; the local coldness and discoloration of the skin after amputation of digits and many other frequently recorded observations of reflexes implicating the sympathetic nerves might be cited. A case in point was that of a physician who had suffered from vascular disturbances involving the right leg for more than a year. His principal complaint was local pain and tenderness in his heel associated with intermittent claudication. If he did not heed the warning cramps that came on with exercise the entire extremity would become ischemic and very painful. At such times it was apparent that the major blood vessels of the leg were no longer pulsating. On the inner side of his right heel was a very tender spot. When this trigger point was pressed upon the pulsations of both the posterior tibial and dorsalis pedis arteries immediately disappeared. If the applied pressure was extreme the return of normal circulation might be delayed for hours.

A recent study of the phantom limb pain syndrome that sometimes follows amputation of a limb has further convinced me that the sympathetic nerves may be involved secondary to nerve fiber irritation. The injection of procaine solution in the region of the sympathetic ganglia from the second to the sixth or seventh thoracic levels causes a prompt alleviation of the pain in many instances and this relief is attended by a remarkable sequence of subjective changes in the phantom limb. The beneficial effects of the single injection sometimes persist for weeks or months and repeated injections may permanently relieve the syndrome. The results obtained by this treatment naturally suggest that afferent impulses of pain have been interrupted by the injections. But such a simple explanation may not be consistent with the facts. Most of the evidence based on anatomical and physiological investigations indicates that the afferent impulses of pain from an extremity do *not* traverse the sympathetic ganglia to reach the spinal cord. If these investigations are accepted at their face value it becomes very difficult to explain satisfactorily the benefits conferred by the procaine injections. However, though the exact mechanism remains obscure, it is increasingly clear that the sympathetic nerves are involved in the pain phenomena of the phantom limb pain syndrome, causalgia and the post-traumatic syndrome, all of which are probably dependent upon irritation of peripheral nerves.

Fourth, may the somatic motor nerves become involved in disturbances dependent upon reflexes arising from local injury?

Certainly pain from a local injury can inhibit the action of voluntary muscles and this in itself is a form of reflex originating from injury. It is also conceivable that afferent impulses from an irritative focus, which are not in themselves painful, may inhibit the somatic motor nerves. I have tried to determine in patients with marked reduction of muscle strength whether or not it was pain that inhibited their response. About all that one can say on this point is that many patients did not complain of pain of any degree when carrying out such tests, and that following the injection of the trigger point or the sympathetic ganglia there was sometimes a prompt increase in the muscle strength.

But the involvement of the voluntary muscles is not confined to loss of strength. In these cases the muscles may show varying degrees of involuntary spasm, be sensitive to direct pressure, and may shorten to a degree that makes tendons prominent and alters the posture of the digits. There is also observed a tendency for the muscles to fibrillate or to jerk periodically as if the neuromuscular mechanism were in a state of heightened irritability.

Fifth, is the spinal cord ever involved in a disturbed physiology by reiterated stimuli from peripheral lesions?

These cases suggest that in addition to local reflexes, some of which must be completed by way of the spinal cord, there may occur changes involving the cord itself. In no other way does it seem reasonable to explain the occurrence of what I have called "mirror images" of the original trouble in the contralateral limb. The instances in which I have observed similar transfer of symptoms to the "normal" side is not confined to this series of cases. Often the pains are ascribed to exactly the same digits on the two sides. The pain may be considerably less severe than on the side of the original injury, but in Case 1 the symptoms involving the "normal" limb were severe enough to lead the patient to request another operation. And the fact that this request was made more than a year after the pain from his original lesion had disappeared would suggest that some organic change had taken place in a segment of the spinal cord. At least it would imply that some physiological disturbance or lowered threshold to pain might persist for long periods of time after the original stimulus is gone. Such a possibility is intriguing because it suggests that the original irritative lesion may so profoundly disturb the normal physiology of the central nervous system that this secondary disturbed function may acquire a momentum of its own which permits it to continue even after the original stimulus has been removed.

It is further possible that the involvement of the spinal cord may not remain confined to a single segment. I have examined two cases that showed objective evidences of swelling and vasomotor alterations to support their claims of subjective complaints in the ipsilateral limb. That several cord segments may be involved is also suggested by the frequent association of "referred" pains felt at a distance from the original lesion and in the distribution of nerves related to different cord levels than the one primarily affected. That these referred pains are directly related to the original lesion appears probable since they may disappear when the trigger point is excised or anesthetized with procaine solution. Steindler has made some interesting observations bearing on this point.

The paroxysms of pain that occur in several of the cases further suggest that the central nervous system may be involved. The premonitory sensations of increasing numbness and the periodicity of the attacks seem to indicate that there is a summation of afferent impulses that finally breaks over the pain threshold. I have noted that sufferers from typical causalgia sometimes deliberately carry out some maneuver to precipitate pain attacks, knowing that a period of relative relief will follow. In a similar manner patients with trigeminal neuralgia may make rapid chewing movements of the jaws before attempting to eat solid food, anticipating that the series of attacks so produced will be followed by a short interval of relief in which they may enjoy their meal. All of these observations suggest that some central mechanism not only summates afferent impulses but also may become temporarily fatigued following a series of discharges.

Whether or not centers higher than the spinal cord may become directly involved in reflex disturbances originating in a trigger point, I shall not attempt to decide. That a constant bombardment of pain impulses may hypersensitize the individual, seems clear enough. Tremor, sweating, rapid pulse, indigestion, disturbances of vision, etc., so frequently accompanying long-continued pain phenomena, may conceivably be the result of reflex involvement of higher centers, or may be only indirectly related to the original lesion and directly related to emotional disturbances secondary to the long continued pain.

Editor's Note: For text discussion, see Chapter 11, p. 90.

Appendix B

The Pain Project Team

James M. Brookhart	USA
Walter Coppock	USA
John K. Friend	USA
Karl-Erik Hagbarth	Sweden
Frederick P. Haugen	USA
Raul Hernández-Péon	Mexico
Margaret A. Kennard	USA
David I.B. Kerr	Australia
Ronald Melzack	Canada
Clare Peterson	USA
Jay Stevens	USA
William A. Stotler	USA

Editor's Note: In the original manuscript the author refers to an appendix with a list of publications by members of the Pain Project team at the University of Oregon. This appendix was not with the material given to us. The reader is referred to Dr. Livingston's earlier books, which probably contain some of these references.

Livingston WK. *Clinical Aspects of Visceral Neurology,* Springfield, IL: Charles Thomas, 1935.

Livingston WK. *Pain Mechanisms,* New York: Macmillan, 1943.

Appendix C

Central Gray Matter
Stimulation in the Monkey

A stimulating electrode was permanently implanted in the central gray matter of a monkey's midbrain. When this area was stimulated the animal gave unmistakable signs that it "disliked" the effects of the stimulus. However, the aim of this experiment was to determine the lowest possible parameters of stimulation that could modify the monkey's behavior. This experiment was difficult to conduct because monkeys are notoriously erratic in their behavior. We devised the following experiment to establish a baseline for such testing. We built a vending machine that required the monkey to press a lever a certain number of times to make the machine deliver a single raisin or peanut. If the machine was set so that 100 lever presses delivered only one reward, the monkey would go to work on the lever, pressing it some 6000 times per hour for perhaps a six-hour period, if it was hungry. We then used this rate as a baseline for behavior under normal circumstances. The monkey could be tested by a single threshold shock of measured intensity and duration to see if the rate of lever pressing was altered. Shocks of remarkably low intensity produced a clearcut falling off of the lever pressing rate that often extended over quite a period of time before the baseline rate was reestablished. If the intensity or duration were slightly raised the monkey often would retreat to the back of his cage after the single shock and would keep away from the lever for some time, even if he was hungry. When he did finally return, he would tentatively press the lever a few times as if trying to see whether it was "safe" to resume the pressing; if he received no additional shocks he would soon be back working the lever at his usual rate.

Editor's Note: This discussion concluded Chapter 21 in the original manuscript.

Appendix D

On comes it now!—The BLAST-OFF—and here we go—to relax for a few moments in a state of weightless speculation. During this brief flight, I am supposed to amuse you by pointing out a few points of interest over which we will pass. We will be much too high to see any details, but we hope that when the retro-rockets have been fired, our heat shield of common sense will protect us during reentry and we will return safely to solid ground.

Down there is Australia. I happen to have a slide taken in Professor Wright's laboratory in Melbourne that shows an adrenalectomized sheep with a parotid fistula from which salivary secretion is dripping slowly into a bucket. As we pass the oat bin, we rattle the dipper against the side of the bin, as if we intended to feed the animal. We do not feed it but we notice a sudden change in its salivary secretion as the drip changes instantly to a steady stream that squirts into the bucket like a tiny hose. But something else about this animal is much more interesting. Before it are three pails, one containing plain water, another containing a very weak water solution of sodium chloride, and a third containing a weak solution of sodium carbonate. All three look alike and presumably would taste alike, but the sheep drinks exclusively from the third pail. Why? We happen to know that the sodium carbonate supplies the sodium need of this animal better than do the fluids in the other two pails, but how does the sheep know it?

Editor's Note: These paragraphs served as a conclusion to the original manuscript. Livingston refers to slides that did not accompany the manuscript we received.

Here is another slide illustrating the same problem. It was taken in Richter's laboratory and it shows several rats, each having some particular dietary deficiency. Each exhibits an uncanny judgment in selecting, from an array of diets, the one best suited to its body needs. Here we see a parathyroidectomized rat that ingests abnormally large amounts of calcium and extremely small amounts of phosphorus. Of course, you will say that the loss of the parathyroid glands has upset the calcium-phosphorus balance in this animal, but what does a rat know about calcium and phosphorus?

Here is a very old slide showing one of Goltz's dogs that had had its neuraxis severed at a particular level. The peculiar thing about this dog is that it is easily aroused to a state of "rage" but it does not follow up its attack in a purposeful way and the manifestations of rage quickly vanish. The animal's behavior seems to lack "conviction" and the observer wonders whether there was any feeling of anger behind it or whether the response was as automatic as the jerking of a monkey on a stick. Later, Bard conducted his classical studies of the "sham rage" to determine just what parts of the brain must be left intact for that state to develop. But, take a look at this picture of one of MacLean's cats, which is in a sustained state of spitting rage that is purposefully directed and sustained. This state has been induced by depositing a minute amount of chemical in the central gray matter of its midbrain (incidentally an area in which responses to tooth-pulp stimulation were found to ascend). While the effect of this chemical persists, it is dangerous to approach this cat, for it will attack viciously anyone who might dare approach it. This state is no "sham rage," no automatic response to a stimulus, but the "real thing."

Here is a picture of Delgado's colony of monkeys, whose behavior he can manipulate by remote control by directly stimulating parts of their "appetitive" systems. Through this control he can make an animal suddenly stop whatever it may be doing and attack a companion as if in rage, or cower as if in fright, eat as if voraciously hungry, or act as if seized with an uncontrollable sexual urge. The boss-bully of this colony, Ali, dominates its behavior but the other monkeys, who have been taught to fear him, now learn that by pressing a lever they can reduce Ali to a docile and submissive companion. What fun!

In all the slides we have seen up to this time we have been observing animal behavior that might or might not be automatic or what we have previously called "instinctual," and we have no way of knowing what the animal may be feeling. But here in the last slide we see some of Heath's human patients, similarly responding to direct brain stimulation. Depending on the stimulation of the stimulating electrode, a patient may be rescued from a psychotic state of rage into a dreamy euphoria or have his behavior altered in many of the patterns exhibited by Delgado's monkeys. But these patients, although far from normal test subjects, usually are able to verbalize their subjective experiences and can describe them as pain, fear, anger, frustration, malaise, happiness, or sexual ecstasy. These are psychotic patients, all of whom are bedeviled by anxieties and abnormal emotional states, some of whom derive a certain degree of relief from self-stimulation. When provided with a set of two or three buttons that they wear in their belts, they can selectively press the one that produced the feelings that best counteract their mental sufferings.

In all the slides I have shown you during this flight we have seen behavioral changes in animals that we can attribute to "conditioning," "instinct," "drive," or an activation of some "appetitive" system. But not until we dealt with human subjects were we able to tell whether the behavior was associated with the appropriate emotion or feeling or might be purely automatic. As we review these slides they may remind us of the 1954 discovery by Olds and Milner of what they thought was a "center" for pleasure and of Delgado's discovery of "three centers for pain."

I have taken you through this thought experiment because I promised to speculate about the possible future of our evolving idea and to register my belief that we are not yet in a position to state with assurance what the essential nature of pain may be. This story has been told in a light-hearted manner but I am serious in my use of the simile of the blind man and the elephant. Our groping hands have palpated only part of the beast and if we would understand him so that we might use this knowledge in our efforts to relieve human suffering, we must know a lot more about him than we do now. For I would say with Polybius, "While a part may conceivably offer a hint of the whole, it cannot possibly yield an exact and certain knowledge of it."

Bibliography

Adair FE, Pack GT, Nicholson, ME. Mélanomes sous-unguéaux et leur diagnostic différencial; à propos de quatre cas. *Bull de l'Ass Franc p. L'Étude du Cancer* 1930; 19:549–566.

Adson AW, Rowntree LG. The surgical indications for sympathetic ganglionectomy and trunk resection in the treatment of chronic arthritis. *Surg Gynecol Obstet* 1930; 50:204–215.

Adson AW. The surgical indications for sympathetic ganglionectomy and trunk resection in the treatment of diseases resulting from vasomotor spasm of peripheral arteries. *Bull NY Acad Med* 1930; 6:17–32.

Alexander W. *The Treatment of Epilepsy.* Edinburgh: Young J. Pentland, 1889.

Allen WF. Formatio reticularis and reticulo-spinal tracts, their visceral functions and possible relationship to tonicity and chronic contractions. *J Wash Acad Sci* 1932; 22:490–495.

Bailey P, Davis EW. Effects of lesions of periaqueductal gray matter on *Macaca mulatta. J Neuropathol Exp Neurol* 1944; 3:69–72.

Barron DH, Matthews BHC. The interpretation of potential changes in the spinal cord. *J Physiol* (Lond) 1938; 92:276–321.

Bernard C. Influence du grand sympathique sur la sensibilité et sur la calorification. *CR Séances Soc Biol Fil* (Paris) 1851; 2:163–164.

Blix M. Experimentelle Beiträge zur Lösung der Frage über die spezifische Energie der Hautnerven. *Ztschr f Biol*, München, 1885, n. F., iii, 145–160.

Bremer F. Cerveau isolé et physiologie du sommeil. *CR Séances Soc Biol Fil* (Paris) 1935; 118:1235–1242.

Burget GE, Livingston WK. The pathway for visceral afferent impulses from forelimb of the dog. *Am J Physiol* 1931; 97:249–253.

Coghill GA. *Anatomy and the Problem of Behavior.* Cambridge: Cambridge University Press, 1929.

Craig W McK. Sympathectomy in the treatment of various diseases. *Am J Nurs* 1931; 31:531–537.

Delgado JMR, Roberts WW, Miller NE. Learning motivated by electrical stimulation of the brain. *Am J Physiol* 1954; 179:587–593.

Dusser de Barenne JG, Ward AA Jr. Reflex inhibition of the knee-jerk from intestinal organs. *Am J Physiol* 1937; 120:340–344.

Dusser de Barenne JG. L'Influence du système nerveux autonome sur la sensibilité de la peau. *J de Psychol* 1931; 28:177–182.

Echlin G, Propper N. Sensitization by injury of the cutaneous nerves in the frog. *J Physiol* 1937; 88:388–400.

Eisenstein EM, Cohen MJ. Learning in an isolated prothoracic insect ganglion. *Animal Behavior* 1965; 13:104–108.

Galambos R. Electrical correlates of learning. In: Brazier MAB (Ed). *CNS and Behavior.* New York: Josiah Macy Jr. Foundation, 1959.

Gaskell WH. *The Involuntary Nervous System.* London, New York: Longmans Green, 1916.

Gellhorn E, Gellhorn H, Trainor J. The influence of spinal irradiations on cutaneous sensations. I. The localization of pain and touch sensations under irradiation. *Am J Physiol* 1931; 97:491–499.

Goldscheider AL. Neue Thatsachen über die Hautsinnesnerven. *Arch f Physiol Leipz* 1885 (Suppl 1–110); p 5.

Granit R, Skoglund CR. Facilitation, inhibition and depression at the "artificial synapse" formed by the cut end of a mammalian nerve. *J Physiol* (Lond) 1945; 103:435–448.

Hagbarth KE, Kerr DIB. Central influences on spinal afferent conduction. *J Neurophysiol* 1954; 17:295–307.

Head H. On disturbances of sensation with especial reference to the pain of visceral disease. *Brain* 1893; 16:1–132.

Head H. *Studies in Neurology,* Vol. 2. Oxford: Oxford University Press, 1920.

Heath RG, Mickle WA. Evaluation of 7 years' experience with depth electrode studies in human patients. In: ER Ramey, DS O'Doherty (Eds). *Electrical Studies on the Unanesthetized Brain.* New York: Hoeber, 1960, pp 214–247.

Hernández-Peón R, Scherrer H, Jouvet M. Modification of electrical activity in cochlear nucleus during "attention" in unanesthetized cats. *Science* 1956; 123:331–332.

Herrick CJ. *The Evolution of Human Nature.* Evanston: University of Texas Press, 1956.

Hopf, M. Über Tumoren des neuromyoarteriellen Glomus (Masson). Frankfurt: *Ztschr f Pathol* 40:387–399, 1930.

Horridge GA. Learning of leg position by headless insects. *Nature* 1962; 193:697–698.

Hurst A. *The Goulstonian Lectures on the Sensibility of the Alimentary Canal.* London: H. Froude and Hodder and Sloughton, 1911.

Jaboulay M. Chirurgie des centres nerveaux, des viscères, et des membres, 2ème vol. Paris: O. Doin, 1902.

Jonnesco T. Angine de poitrine guérie par la résection du sympathétique cervico-thoracique. *Bull Acad Natl Med* (Paris) 1920; 84:93–102.

Keele KD. *Anatomies of Pain.* Oxford: Blackwell, 1957.

Kennard MA. Sensitization of the spinal cord of the cat to pain-inducing stimuli. *J Neurosurg* 1953; 10:169–177.

Kopeloff LM, Chusid JG, Kopeloff N. Epilepsy in *Macaca mulatta* after cortical or intracerebral alumina. *Arch Neurol Psychiatr* 1955; 74:523–526

Kramer JG, Todd TW. The distribution of nerves to the arteries of the arm, with a discussion of the clinical value of results. *Anat Rec* 1914; 8:243–255.

Langley JN. *The Autonomic Nervous System.* Cambridge: Heffer, 1921.

Lashley KS. *Brain Mechanisms and Intelligence.* Chicago: University of Chicago Press, 1929.

Lennander KG. Beobachtungen über die Sensibilität in der Bauchhöhle. *Mitteilungen aus den Grenzgebieten der Medizin und Chirurgie* 1902; 10:38–104.

Leriche, René. De l'élongation et de la section des nerfs périvasculaires dans certains syndromes douloureux d'origine artérielle et dans quelques troubles trophiques. *Lyon Chirurgical* 1913; 10:378–382.

Leriche, René. De la causalgie envisagée comme une névrite du sympathique et de son traitement par la dénudation et l'excision des plexus nerveux péri-artériels. *Presse Med* 1916; 24:178–180.

Lewis T. *Pain*. New York: Macmillan, 1942, pp 68–83.

Lewis T. The nocifensor system of nerves and its reactions. *Br Med J* 1937; 1:431–435.

Lilly JC. Learning motivated by subcortical stimulation: the "start" and "stop" patterns of behavior. In: HH Jasper (Ed). *Reticular Formation of the Brain*. Boston: Little Brown, 1958.

Livingston WK. *Pain Mechanisms*. New York: Macmillan, 1943.

Livingston WK. *Clinical Aspects of Visceral Neurology*. Springfield, Illinois: Charles Thomas, 1935.

Livingston WK. Post-traumatic pain syndromes: an interpretation of the underlying pathological physiology, Div I. *West J Surg Obstet Gynecol* 1938a; 46:341–347.

Livingston WK. Post-traumatic pain syndromes: an interpretation of the underlying pathological physiology, Div II. *West J Surg Obstet Gynecol* 1938b; 46:426–434.

MacKenzie J. Some points bearing on the association of sensory disorders and visceral disease. *Brain* 1893; 16:321–354.

MacKenzie J Sir. *Angina Pectoris*. London: H. Froude and Hodder and Stoughton, 1923.

MacKenzie J. *Symptoms and Their Interpretation*. London: Shaw & Sons, 1909.

Magoun HW. *The Waking Brain*, 2nd ed. Springfield: Charles Thomas, 1963, pp 116–128.

Masson P. Le glomus neuromyoartériel des régions tactiles et ses tumeurs. *Lyon Chirurgical* 1924; 21:257–280.

Mitchell SW. *Injuries of Nerves and Their Consequences*. Philadelphia: Lippincott, 1872.

Morruzzi G, Magoun HW. Brain stem reticular formation and activation of the EEG. *EEG Clin Neurophysiol* 1949; 1:455–473.

Müller J. *Elements of Physiology*, vol 2, translated from the German by Wm. Baly, arranged from the 2nd London edition by John Bell. Philadelphia: Lea and Blanchard, 1843.

Odermatt W. Die Schmerzempfindlichkeit der Blutgefäße und die Gefäßreflexe. Tübingen: *Beiträge zur Klinischen Chirurgie*, 1922; 12:1–84.

Olds J, Milner P. Positive reinforcement produced by electrical stimulation of septal area and other regions of rat brain. *J Comp Physiol Psychol* 1954; 47:419–427.

Olds ME, Olds J. Approach-avoidance analysis of rat diencephalon. *J Comp Neurol* 1963; 120:259–295.

Paré A. *Les œuvres d'Ambroise Paré*. Paris: Gabriel Buon, 1598. (Histoire du défunct Roy Charles IX, *10th Book*, Chap 41, p 401) Quoted in Livingston WK. *Pain Mechanisms*. New York: Macmillan, 1943.

Pollock LJ, Davis LE. *Peripheral Nerve Injuries*. New York: Paul Hoeber, 1933.

Ross J. On the segmental distribution of sensory disorders. *Brain* 1888; 10:333–361.

Royle ND. Treatment of spastic paralysis by sympathetic ramisection. *Proc R Soc Med* (Sect Orthop) 1927; 20:63–68.

Sem-Jacobsen CW. *Depth-electrographic Stimulation of the Human Brain and Behavior: From Fourteen Years of Studies and Treatment of Parkinson's Disease and Mental Disorders with Implanted Electrodes.* Springfield, Illinois: Charles Thomas, 1968.

Sharpless S, Jasper HH. Habituation of the arousal reaction. *Brain* 1956; 79:655–680.

Speranskii AD. *A Basis for the Theory of Medicine.* CP Dutt, AS Sukkov (Trans, Eds). New York: International Publishers, 1936.

Sperry RW. Brain bisection and mechanisms of consciousness. In: UC Eccles (Ed). *Brain and Conscious Experience.* Berlin: Springer-Verlag, 1966, pp 298–308.

Tinel J. Causalgie du nerf médian par blessure à la partie moyenne du bras; insuffisance de la sympathectomie périartérielle; guérison par la section du nerf au poignet. *Rev Neurol* Paris 1918; 25:79–82.

Tönnies JF. Reflex discharge from the spinal cord over the posterior roots. *J Neurophysiol* 1938; 1:378–390.

von Frey M. *Berichte über die Verhandlungen der k. Sächsischen Gesellschaft der Wissenschaften.* Leipzig: bei S. Hirzel, 1894; 185–196; and 1985; p 166.

Walker AE, Kollros JJ, Case TJ. Physiological basis of concussion. *J Neurosurg* 1944; 1:103–116.

Woollard HH. Anatomy of peripheral sensation. *Br Med J* 1936; 2:861–862.

Index